NCLEX

LAB VALUES

74 Must Know Lab Values to Help
You Survive Nursing School and Kick-
Ass on the NCLEX

100+ NCLEX Practice Questions and
Rationales

Chris Mulder, CRNA, MSN

Contents

About the Author

My name is Chris Mulder, a full-time nurse anesthetist at a level 1 trauma center in Central Florida. Long before becoming a CRNA, I worked in a tiny cubicle all day in a position that rendered my English degree useless. That only lasted a couple of years before I realized something had to change before I lost my mind. Much to my wife's dismay, I decided to go back to school to get my nursing degree. It wasn't easy, but I made it through. After graduation, I worked as a registered nurse in the medical ICU in a large hospital in Lakeland, FL. A few years later, I applied for Nurse Anesthesia School, and the rest is history!

As I've gone through my years of training and working as a nurse, I've come to realize a few things. The information I was getting in the classroom was difficult to retain and rarely translated to real-world practice. I also found that most nurses took themselves too seriously and were often condescending. That's why I try to keep things a little more light-hearted without all the arrogance.

I know what you're going through. I remember the constant struggle and the sleepless nights. I know the butterflies in the stomach before clinicals and the sinking feeling right before submitting an exam. Stick with me and we'll get through this together. I might be a nurse anesthetist, but I am a NURSE before anything else.

Introduction

Getting lab values down is an important nursing skill that we all must learn how to master. The problem is that most books drown you in information that makes it nearly impossible to remember. I tried to organize this book in a concise way that keeps out all the fluff. So if you're looking for a detailed in-depth description of every possible lab value, then this probably isn't for you. These are some of the most common labs with the most relevant information, written in a way you can understand.

The labs are organized in alphabetical order, but each of them can be accessed quickly by clicking in the table of contents. Each lab includes the most common reasons they are drawn, the normal value range, and a brief description. Some are longer than others, as I sometimes felt the need to include more information for certain topics. Put it this way...it wouldn't be on the page if I didn't think it was important.

I have also included a helpful mnemonic for each lab. Almost all of them I came up with myself to help me get through nursing school. Because of this, some of them are pretty silly and might not be for you. If they help, use them. If not, no big deal. You can even try to come up with some on your own. It's not difficult, and the simple process of creating them can help you remember the information. Keep in mind that every lab in this book assumes an adult patient, and that the value may be different for children.

After reviewing the labs, try some of the 110 NCLEX-style practice questions! If you'd like to skip the content review and go straight for the questions, feel free to skip ahead to page 153.

Acid-Fast Bacillus (AFB)

- **Purpose**: Diagnose Tuberculosis (TB)

- **Mnemonic**: "Get an AFB to help you diagnose TB"

- **Normal**: Negative

AFB Smear
- This is a smear typically taken from a sputum sample that can reveal if there is any mycobacteria present. Mycobacteria are types of bacteria that cause a number of different infections, such as tuberculosis. If the smear comes back positive, then you'll know that there is a chance that your patient has TB. However, this is not a definitive diagnosis, as mycobacteria can also cause other infections, such as Leprosy. But it is a quick way to determine if your patient should be placed on isolation and what kind of treatment should be started. Although other body fluids can be tested, the most common is sputum. The results from this type of test can usually be seen within a few hours.

AFB Culture
- Because this test is much more sensitive, it can usually confirm a diagnosis of

tuberculosis. It will tell you if any mycobacteria is found, and if so, what type it is. If no mycobacteria is found, then your patient's symptoms are from something else. Because the test is so specific, it takes much longer than an AFB smear, as long as 6-8 weeks. If a patient has had tuberculosis in the past, this test can also help to determine if it is active or not.

Activated Clotting Time (ACT)

- **Purpose**: 1. Liver function, 2. Heparin Therapy

- **Mnemonic**: "Check the A C T on Heparin therapy"
  "When your liver is jacked, you'll increase the ACT"

- **Normal**: 70-120 Seconds
  Therapeutic: 150-600 Seconds

- **Increased**: Heparin, Liver Disease, Coumadin, Clotting Disorders
- **Decreased**: Thrombosis

The ACT is measured in seconds, and is typically used when a patient is on heparin therapy to see how effective it is. It tells you how long the blood takes to clot. An ACT of 200 seconds tells you that it took 200 seconds for the blood to clot. The larger the number, the more anticoagulated the patient is. A certain therapeutic range is aimed for, and the ACT can help guide the titration of heparin.

The therapeutic goal varies, depending on the reason for anticoagulation. For example, you typically want your ACT to be above 400-480 during cardiopulmonary bypass. Other tests, such as a Partial Thromboplastin Time (PTT), can also evaluate the effectiveness of heparin. However, most of these tests take much longer to get back than an ACT, which can be read on a portable machine in real-time.

Heparin is not the only thing that will cause an increase in the ACT. You might also see this when there is liver damage, the patient is on Coumadin, or there is a deficiency in clotting factors. It can even be increased somewhat if the patient is hypothermic.

You might see a decrease when there is thrombosis.

Adrenocorticotropic Hormone (ACTH)

- **Purpose**: Diagnose Addison Disease and Cushing Syndrome

- **Mnemonic**: "Addison/Cushing Test Hormone"

- **Normal** (varies by time of day):
  - AM: 10-60 pg/mL (2.2 – 13.3 pmol/L)
  - PM: 5-20 pg/mL (1.1 – 4.5 pmol/L)

- **Increased**: Addison Disease, Cushing Syndrome/Disease, Stress
- **Decreased**: Adrenal Adenoma, Cushing Syndrome, Steroids, Secondary Adrenal Insufficiency, Hypopituitarism

The ACTH measures the function of the anterior pituitary gland. Corticotropin-releasing hormone (CRH) comes from the hypothalamus and causes ACTH to be released from the anterior pituitary. Once this happens, the ACTH causes cortisol production from the adrenal cortex. I know your eyes may be glazing over by now, but try to bear with me.

Hypothalamus -> CRH -> Anterior Pituitary -> ACTH -> Adrenal Cortex -> Cortisol

- Cushing Syndrome/Disease:

  Cushing *Syndrome* is an umbrella term meaning that there is *too much cortisol* being produced. Cushing *Disease* means that the reason for the increase is specifically due to a pituitary tumor causing ACTH release. If the reason for the increase is a non-pituitary (ectopic) tumor, then it would fall only under the Cushing Syndrome definition. These are often in the pancreas, thymus, lungs, or ovaries. A high cortisol level with an ACTH level below normal usually means that the cause is an adrenal adenoma.

  Increased Cortisol + *Increased* ACTH = Pituitary Tumor (Cushing Disease)
  or
  Non-Pituitary Tumor (Cushing Syndrome only)

  Increased Cortisol + *Decreased* ACTH = Adrenal Adenoma (Cushing Syndrome only)

- Addison Disease:

  The problem in someone with Addison Disease is that there is *not enough cortisol* being produced. Again, there are 2 possible causes: either there is primary adrenal gland failure or the patient has hypopituitarism. If the ACTH is increased, it typically means that the problem is coming from the adrenal gland. This happens sometimes during infarction or hemorrhage. It can also happen if the adrenal gland has been removed, or if there is adrenal suppression after chronic steroid use. If the ACTH is low, then the most common cause is hypopituitarism, which just means that there is not enough secretion of ACTH from the pituitary.

Decreased Cortisol + *Increased* ACTH = Primary Addison
Decreased Cortisol + *Decreased* ACTH = Hypopituitarism

*Make note of the fact that normal ACTH levels change throughout the day. They are typically higher in the morning, and decrease as the day goes on. Because of this variation, labs are usually taken in the morning (before 8am).

Alanine Aminotransferase (ALT, SGPT)

- **Purpose**: Liver Function

- **Mnemonic**: "Awful Liver Trouble"

- **Normal**: 4 – 36 Units/L

- **Increased**: Liver Disease, Shock, Trauma, Burns, MI, Pancreatitis

ALT is a substance found in a few different places in the body, but is most highly concentrated in the liver. Anytime there is damage to the liver, ALT is released. The ALT is usually taken at the same time as the AST (aspartate aminotransferase) in a comprehensive metabolic panel. It is also included with the other LFTs (Liver Function Tests) in a hepatic panel. These often include the PT/INR, PTT, Albumin, and Bilirubin. The ratio of AST to ALT will typically be above 1.0 in chronic liver conditions, and below 1.0 in more acute problems.

Albumin

- **Purpose**: 1. Liver Function, 2. Determine Nutrition Status, 3. Determine Fluid Status

- **Mnemonic**:
  - ➤ "If the albumin is high, then your patient is dry"
  - ➤ "If the albumin is low, then your liver is slow"

- **Normal**: 3.5-5 g/dL (35-50 g/L)

- **Increased**: Certain Medications, Dehydration
- **Decreased**: Kidney Disease, Liver Disease, Malnutrition, Celiac Disease, Chron's Disease,
  Pregnancy

Albumin, along with globulin, makes up most of the total protein in the body. Sometimes, total protein is referred to when determining if a patient's albumin is low. Normal total protein in an adult is 6.4-8.3 g/dL.

Albumin is the largest component of the total protein in the blood. It is produced in the liver and its job is to maintain the colloidal osmotic pressure. This pressure makes sure that fluid is balanced between the tissues in the body and the capillaries. Normally, it is inclined to pull water into the capillaries. When there is a problem, water can leak out into the tissue, causing edema.

Some examples of problems causing low albumin include malnutrition, liver disease, and severe burns. It is also common to have a decreased albumin in late pregnancy. If your patient's albumin is low, it can be replaced via IV. But the underlying cause will need to be addressed, or it will keep dropping. Albumin may be increased when a patient is dehydrated. However, dehydration is typically a fairly easy thing to diagnose, so an albumin level is not normally needed.

Alkaline Phosphatase (ALP, Alk Phos)

- **Purpose**: 1. Liver Function, 2. Bone Growth

- **Mnemonic**:
  - ➢ "ALP means there is A Liver Problem"
  - ➢ "When there's more Alk Phos, check for increased Oss (Osseus/Bone)"

- **Normal**: 30-120 units/L (Adults)

- **Increased**: Liver Disease, Paget Disease, Rickets, Sarcoidosis, Hyperparathyroidism, Growing Bone
- **Decreased**: Hypothyroidism, Celiac Disease, Scurvy, Malnutrition, Pernicious Anemia, Too Much B12 in Diet

ALP is a substance found in many places throughout the body, but it's mostly contained in the bone, liver, and biliary tract. This lab is drawn when you want to diagnose disorders in these areas. The types of liver dysfunction that increase ALP the most include cirrhosis, obstructive biliary disease, and metastatic tumors.

ALP is also increased more when there is new bone growth. Because of this, you will see a higher level in kids and teenagers. There is also new abnormal bone growth when there is metastasis to the bone, fractures that are healing, rheumatoid arthritis, Paget disease, and hyperparathyroidism.

Ammonia

- **Purpose**: Liver Function

- **Mnemonic**: "If your patient's in a coma, check the ammonia"

- **Normal**: 10-80 mcg/dL (Adult)

- **Increased**: Liver Disease, Reye's Syndrome, Heart Failure, Hepatic Encephalopathy
- **Decreased**: Hypertension

When a patient has severe liver problems, such as cirrhosis or hepatitis, ammonia levels can increase to dangerous levels. Proteins in the body are broken down into ammonia, among other things. Ammonia then goes to the liver, which converts it into urea. The urea then goes to the kidneys and is banished from the body through the urine. This process keep everything status quo.

When there are liver problems, this process is disrupted, and ammonia is allowed to simply run wild. This is not good, as it easily makes its way to the brain, causing hepatic encephalopathy. The patient might start out being confused and disoriented. If the ammonia levels continue to rise, it may eventually lead to a coma.

Lactulose is a medication that be given orally or rectally to help bring down these high levels. The ammonia can then be removed by way of the colon. If you give your patient this, be prepared for a long night! This is obviously not a cure, however, as you will need to correct the underlying cause.

Amylase

- **Purpose**: Pancreas Function

- **Mnemonic**: "Amylase and Lipase tell you about the Pancreas(e)"

- **Normal**: 30-220 units/L

- **Increased**: Pancreatitis, Mumps, Rheumatoid Disease, DKA, Severe Peptic Ulcers, Necrotic Bowel, Ectopic Pregnancy

Amylase is a substance that is secreted from something called pancreatic acinar cells. It then goes into the pancreatic duct before entering the duodenum. Once in the small intestine, amylase breaks down carbohydrates until they become simple sugars. Check it out:

Acinar Cells -> Amylase -> Pancreatic Duct -> Duodenum

If there is damage to the acinar cells or the duct, then amylase starts pouring out at a much higher rate. This extra amylase is absorbed into the blood stream and shows up on the lab result. Persistent problems, such as pancreatitis or pancreatic cancer, will cause these levels to remain high.

Although an increased level of amylase will usually show signs of pancreatic problems, there are other things that could cause it as well. For example, high levels can also be seen with a bowel obstruction, mumps, ectopic pregnancy, and severe DKA (diabetic ketoacidosis).

Anion Gap (AG)

- **Purpose**: Determine Level of Acidity

- **Mnemonic**: "Anion Gap = Acidosis Guide"

- **Normal**: 3-11 mEq/L

- **Increased**: Lactic Acidosis, DKA, Renal Failure,
  Starvation

- **Decreased**: Multiple Myeloma, Lithium Toxicity, Low Protein, Excessive Vomiting, Too Much Alkali in the Diet

The anion gap is a measure of the difference between the cations (+) and the anions (-) that are in the extracellular fluid. The higher the number, the more acidotic (+) the blood is. This can happen in a few different cases. For example, if a patient has a bad infection that gets into the bloodstream, they can develop lactic acidosis. Also, diabetic patients may go into ketoacidosis. Patients in renal failure can lose a lot of bicarbonate, while holding on to acids. In each case, the anion gap may increase above normal.

It is possible for the anion gap to be decreased, but it is very unlikely. You might see it drop when the albumin is low or when there are abnormal plasma cells.

There are a couple different equations to determine the anion gap, depending on whether or not the potassium level is included.

<u>Without K</u>:   AG = [Na] – ([Cl] + [HCO3])

<u>With K</u>:   AG = ([Na] + [K]) – ([Cl] + [HCO3])

Antidiuretic Hormone (ADH, Vasopressin)

- **Purpose**:
  - ➢ Diagnose Diabetes Insipidus (DI)
  - ➢ Diagnose Syndrome of Inappropriate ADH Secretion (SIADH)

- **Mnemonic**: "ADH = Absorb Dry H2O"

- **Normal**: 1-5 pg/mL

- **Increased**: SIADH, Nephrogenic Diabetes Insipidus, Dehydration, Trauma
- **Decreased**: Neurogenic Diabetes Insipidus, Hypervolemia, Surgical Cutting of the Pituitary

ADH is produced in the hypothalamus, but gets stored in the posterior pituitary gland. The primary function of ADH is to regulate the volume of water that is pulled back into the body by the kidneys. There are 2 main things that can cause it to be released from the posterior pituitary: a rise in serum osmolality (e.g. dehydration) or a reduction in intravascular blood volume (e.g. hemorrhage).

Let's think this over for a second to let it sink in. If you are dehydrated, your osmolality is high. Imagine a glass of salt water sitting in the sun. As the water evaporates, the ratio of salt to water will begin to increase. The more water that is lost to evaporation, the greater the osmolality becomes of the contents in the glass. More salt plus less water equals a higher osmolality. This is easy to translate back to the body, especially since the two main substances ADH is concerned with are salt (Na) and water (H_2O).

When there is a hemorrhage in the body, the reason for ADH to act is essentially the same: there is decreased intravascular volume. If you lose water or blood, ADH will tell the kidneys to start holding onto more water.

Since the kidneys are reabsorbing more water into the body, less is being excreted into the urine. Because of this, the osmolality of the fluid in the body will start to decrease (more water, less concentrated), while the osmolality of the urine will start to increase (less water, more concentrated).

Low intravascular volume -> Hypothalamus -> Posterior Pituitary -> ADH -> Kidneys

Increased Na + *Decreased* H_2O = *High* Concentration = *High* Osmolality

Decreased Na + *Increased* H_2O = *Low* Concentration = *Low* Osmolality

ADH is constantly secreted to maintain a balance, adjusting with more or less as needed.

Sometimes, there isn't enough ADH secretion to maintain this balance. Sometimes, the kidneys decide to put on their headphones and ignore the message ADH is sending. When either of these things happen, you get Diabetes Insipidus (DI). If the cause for this is lack of ADH secretion, it is likely a problem with the central neurologic system (tumor, trauma, etc). This would be known as neurogenic DI. If the problem is with the kidneys, it is known as nephrogenic DI. In either case, you will see large amounts of diluted urine (Low osmolality) and highly concentrated fluid in the body (High osmolality).

DI = *Decreased* ADH secretion OR *Decreased* Kidney response -> High Blood Osmolality

Sometimes, you know right away if the patient's DI is neurological or nephrogenic. But if you need to find out for sure, you can do the "water deprivation test." Patients are instructed to limit their intake of water and vasopressin (synthetic ADH) is injected. If the patient has neurogenic DI, the urine osmolality will not increase when there is little intake of water, but it will after vasopressin is given. If the patient has nephrogenic DI, urine osmolality will not increase in either case. A blood test can also reveal the cause of DI, as ADH levels are lower when the problem is neurogenic, but higher when the problem is nephrogenic.

Another problem that people often confuse diabetes insipidus with is the syndrome of inappropriate ADH secretion (SIADH). In this case, too much ADH is being secreted. Because of this, the kidneys respond by reabsorbing large amounts of water. This low osmolality in the blood can lead to hyponatremia (Low Na), hypokalemia (Low K), and hypocalcemia (Low Ca), among other things. This can cause major cardiac, neurological, and metabolic problems.

SIADH = Increased ADH secretion -> H2O resorption -> Low Blood Osmolality

Arterial Blood Gas (ABG)

- **Purpose**: Respiratory Function

- **Mnemonic**:
  - ➤ "To find out if the lungs will pass, draw some blood and get a gas"

- **Normal Values:** (see table)

pH	7.35 – 7.45
HCO3	22 – 26 mEq/L
PaO2	80 – 100 mmHg
PaCO2	35 – 45 mmHg
SaO2	95 – 100%
Base Excess	-2 to +2 mEq/L

ABGs can be tricky to learn when you're first starting out. However, once you have the hang of it, it's really pretty simple and becomes second nature. ABGs are obtained by getting a sample of blood from an artery. The main purpose is to see how well the lungs are functioning. If you get blood from a vein instead of an artery, it will have already delivered the oxygenated gas to the rest of the body. This number would not accurately reflect what the lungs had delivered.

The first thing an ABG will tell you is the pH of the blood, followed by all of the factors that helped it get to that number. These factors include the partial pressure of oxygen (PaO2), the partial pressure of carbon dioxide (PaCO2), bicarbonate (HCO3), and Base Excess (BE). It will also tell you the oxygen saturation, which can help to confirm the accuracy of the patient's pulse oximeter.

Take a look at the table to see the reference values. This will help you in determining whether a patient is acidotic or alkalotic and why. The first thing you want to look at is the pH. A low pH (<7.35) tells you that the patient is acidotic, while a high pH (>7.45) tells you that they are alkalotic. The next thing you want to determine is cause of the abnormality, whether it be metabolic or respiratory in nature. CO2 is affected by respiratory conditions, while HCO3 is affected by metabolic conditions.

Respiratory Acidosis = *Low* pH + *High* CO2 + *normal* HCO3
Respiratory Alkalosis = *High* pH + *Low* CO2 + *normal* HCO3
Metabolic Acidosis = *Low* pH + *normal* CO2 + *Low* HCO3
Metabolic Alkalosis = *High* pH + *normal* CO2 + *High* HCO3

So, more CO2 means lower pH, while more HCO3 means a higher pH. Got it? Great! Now let's make it a little more complicated. You can go a step further in this equation by figuring out whether or not the acidosis or alkalosis is compensated or uncompensated. It sounds confusing, but it's a piece of cake. During respiratory acidosis or alkalosis, the kidneys might try to compensate for the problem. It does this by either holding onto HCO_3 (during resp. acidosis), or by getting rid of it (during resp. alkalosis). The Lungs can also try to compensate when the kidneys are causing the pH imbalance. It does this either by holding onto CO_2 (during met. Alkalosis) or by getting rid of it (during met. acidosis). If the pH is corrected to normal, it is considered compensated. If the pH is close to normal, but still out of range, it is considered partially compensated. If the pH is abnormal and it doesn't appear the kidneys or lungs are doing anything about it, then it is considered uncompensated.

Respiratory Acidosis (Compensated) = *Normal* pH + *High* CO_2 + *High* HCO_3 (CO_2 more out of range)

Respiratory Alkalosis (Compensated) = *Normal* pH + *Low* CO_2 + *Low* HCO_3 (CO_2 more out of range)

Metabolic Acidosis (Compensated) = *Normal* pH + *Low* CO_2 + *Low* HCO_3 (HCO_3 more out of range)

Metabolic Alkalosis (Compensated) = *Normal* pH + *High* CO_2 + *High* HCO_3 (HCO_3 more out of range)

Aspartate Aminotransferase (AST, SGOT)

- **Purpose**: Liver Function

- **Mnemonic**: "High <u>AST</u> = n<u>AST</u>y Liver"

- **Normal**: 0 – 35 Units/L

- **Increased**: Liver Disease, Pancreatitis, Certain Anemias, Certain Skeletal Muscle Disorders
- **Decreased**: DKA, Pregnancy, Renal Disease

Whenever there is some suspected problem with the liver, an AST is a standard diagnostic tool that tells you how bad things really are. When the liver gets damaged, AST is released at levels proportional to the damage. So, the more of the liver that is damaged, the higher the AST will be. It takes 8 hours for AST levels to rise, and it is cleared from the body within a few days if there is no further damage. In chronic diseases, such as cirrhosis and hepatitis, the levels will remain high.

The AST is usually taken at the same time as the ALT (alanine aminotransferase), along with the other LFTs (Liver Function Tests). These often include the PT/INR, PTT, Albumin, and Bilirubin.

The ratio of AST to ALT will typically be above 1.0 in chronic liver conditions, and below 1.0 in more acute problems. Other things that may cause a brief increase in AST levels include pancreatitis, trauma, some musculoskeletal disorders, and some renal diseases. You might find a decreased ALT in DKA, pregnancy, and in patients who have been on dialysis.

Atrial Natriuretic Peptide (ANP)

- **Purpose**: Diagnose CHF

- **Mnemonic**: "Against Na and Pressure"

- **Normal**: 22 – 37 pg/mL

- **Increased**: CHF, MI, Hypertension, Rejection of Heart Transplant

Similar to BNP, ANP is a substance that gets sent from the atria in the heart whenever there is an increased amount of blood volume. A typical example of this would be in CHF (Congestive Heart Failure), a condition this test is commonly used for. This main function is to lower the blood volume by decreasing water and sodium, which will eventually cause a decrease in the blood pressure. This is the opposite of the function aldosterone has.

Once ANP is released, it will cause an increase in the GFR (Glomerular Filtration Rate), which allows more sodium and water to be excreted from the body. ANP will also decrease the reabsorption rate of sodium and water back into the body, and will impede renin and aldosterone secretion. Renin and aldosterone are part of the renin-angiotensin-aldosterone system, which is a conversation for another day. For now, just know that this system is inclined to increase water, sodium, and blood pressure. So by inhibiting this, ANP is allowing for a decrease in all of these things. In addition to the renal effects, ANP also causes the vascular smooth muscle to relax, causing a further decrease in blood pressure.

Bilirubin

- **Purpose**: 1. Liver Function, 2. Bile Duct Function

- **Mnemonic**: "Bilirubin = Bile Test"

- **Normal**:
  - Total: 0.3 - 1.0 mg/dL
  - Indirect: 0.2 - 0.8 mg/dL
  - Direct: 0.1 - 0.3 mg/dL

- **Increased**: Gallstones, Liver Disease, Duct Obstruction, Excessive Blood Transfusions, Sepsis, Certain Types of Anemia, Neonatal Hyperbilirubinemia

After hemoglobin gets released from RBCs (red blood cells), it is simplified into heme and globin. The heme eventually becomes bilirubin. This type of bilirubin is considered "Indirect." "Direct" bilirubin comes from the liver when the indirect bilirubin is linked with a substance known as a glucuronide. This direct bilirubin is then sent out to the hepatic ducts, common bile duct, and the bowel. Total bilirubin is the sum of the indirect and direct bilirubin.

Bilirubin makes up a major portion of bile. When the liver has a hard time getting rid of the bilirubin, it begins to build up in the body and can cause jaundice (a yellowish discoloration of the skin). If the reason for the build-up is due to a liver disorder, then the indirect bilirubin will be increased. If the issue lies beyond the liver, as is the case with gallstones and blocked bile ducts, then the direct bilirubin will be increased.

In newborns, the liver is often too immature to convert the indirect bilirubin to direct bilirubin. Because of this, the indirect bilirubin will build up, causing jaundice. This is why you will often see newborn babies with a yellow tint to their skin. This is usually not a problem and will resolve itself within a few days. However, it needs to be monitored and treated if necessary. If the bilirubin level gets too high, it can get to the brain, leading to encephalopathy. If this happens, the infant may be difficult to arouse and can even go into a coma.

Blood Urea Nitrogen (BUN)

- **Purpose**: Kidney Function

- **Mnemonic**: "BUNKBED: High <u>BUN</u> means the <u>K</u>idneys are in <u>BED</u>"

- **Normal**: 3-20 mg/dL

- **Increased**: Kidney Disease, Dehydration, Sepsis, Burns, GI Bleed, CHF, Urinary Tract Obstructions, Certain Meds, Shock
- **Decreased**: Liver Disease, Pregnancy, Malnutrition, Hypervolemia, Nephrotic Syndrome

Urea is produced mostly in the liver before getting dissolved into the blood and excreted by the kidneys (the renal tubules, to be exact). When something in this process isn't working as well, the BUN will increase above normal. Although this can sometimes be caused by liver problems, this lab test is most often used to help diagnose kidney problems. The kidneys are falling asleep instead of doing their job to get rid of that stuff.

With that said, sometimes the problem isn't due to the kidneys or the liver. For example, a high protein diet can elevate the BUN, as can hemorrhage, trauma, and certain medications.

When diagnosing renal disorders, the BUN is looked at in close relation to the creatinine level. This can be seen as the BUN/Creatinine ratio. When the intravascular volume in the body decreases, such as with dehydration, this ratio increases. If the ratio is above 20, then the issue is often coming from something before the kidneys (pre-renal).

Brain Natriuretic Peptide (BNP)

- **Purpose**: Diagnose CHF

- **Mnemonic**: "<u>B</u>locks <u>N</u>a and <u>P</u>ressure"

- **Normal**: < 100 pg/mL

- **Increased**: CHF, MI, Hypertension, Rejection after Heart Transplant

While the Atrial Natriuretic Peptide (ANP) is sent out from the atria of the heart, BNP is sent out from the ventricles. The name "brain natriuretic peptide" is a little confusing. Long ago, BNP was first discovered in the brains of pig cadavers. However, we now know that in humans, it comes mostly from the heart. Unfortunately, in an attempt to complicate nursing students' lives, the name stuck.

This substance is released whenever there is too much stretching of muscles in the heart. This happens in cases such as CHF, a problem this test is often used to diagnose. The main function is to lower the blood volume by decreasing water and sodium, which will eventually cause a decrease in the blood pressure. This is the opposite of the function aldosterone has.

The worse the CHF is, the higher the BNP will rise. It may also be high when patients have had uncontrolled hypertension for a long period of time or in patients who recently had a heart attack (Myocardial Infarction).

BRCA

- **Purpose**: Identify Breast Cancer Risk

- **Mnemonic**: "BReast CAncer" (I didn't come up with this one...BRCA is the actual acronym)

- **Normal**: Negative

The BRCA is a test that can tell you if there is an increased likelihood of developing breast cancer. Often, people who have an increased risk will have this test done, so they can take appropriate steps if needed. Although women are the majority getting this test done, it is also recommended in men who are at risk. BRCA1 and BRCA2 are the genes most often seen with the mutation that suggests an increased breast cancer risk. If one of these mutations are present, over 50% of the time breast cancer develops by age 50. If the test comes back positive, it is usually recommended that prophylactic mastectomies be performed.

C-reactive Protein (CRP)

- **Purpose**: Determine Infection or Inflammation

- **Mnemonic**: "Check for Redness and Puffiness"

- **Normal**: < 1.0 mg/dL

- **Increased**: Arthritis, Bacterial Infection, Chron's Disease, Rheumatic Fever, TB, UTI, Trauma, PE, MI, Lupus, Transplant Rejection

An elevated CRP indicates that there is some kind of bacterial infection or other inflammatory response going on in the body. It is not specific, so it can't tell you exactly what the problem is or where it's coming from. But it can be a good place to start if you don't have anything else to go by. If medications are given to decrease the inflammation, such as steroids, the CRP levels will also decrease.

Many things other than a bacterial infection can cause an increase. You will likely see it rise in any condition that causes inflammation, such as rheumatic fever, myocardial infarction, lupus, trauma, etc. Once the cause of the increase is taken care of, the CRP should return to normal within a few days. Decreased levels are less common, but may be seen after weight loss, exercise, or alcohol intake.

Calcium (Ca)

- **Purpose**: Electrolytes

- **Mnemonic**:
  - ➢ Hypocalcemia Symptoms: "MAST: Muscle Weakness, Arrhythmias, Stridor, Tetany"
  - ➢ Hypercalcemia Symptoms: "CANS: Confusion/Coma, Arrhythmias, Nausea, Stones"

- **Normal**:
  - ➢ Total: 9 - 10.5 mg/dL (2.25-2.75 mmol/L)
  - ➢ Ionized: 4.5 – 6 mg/dL (1.05-1.3 mmol/L)

- **Increased**: Hyperthyroidism, Hyperparathyroidism, Addison Disease, Lymphoma, Paget Disease, Sarcoidosis, TB, Certain Cancers
- **Decreased**: Hypoparathyroidism, Hypoalbuminemia, Alkalosis, Renal Failure, Pancreatitis, Fat Embolism, Vitamin D Deficiency, Rickets, Malabsorption

Total Calcium includes all of the calcium in the blood, including the protein-bound form and ionized form. Calcium that is bound to protein is dependent on that protein, which consists mostly of albumin. Because of this, total calcium can be affected by the patient's albumin level. If the albumin is low, then the calcium won't have as much protein to bind to, and will therefore be lower. A more accurate representation of a patient's calcium level is that in the ionized form, since it is not dependent on anything else.

High calcium (hypercalcemia) can be caused by hyperparathyroidism, too much vitamin D intake, metastasis, tuberculosis, and sarcoidosis. Low calcium (hypocalcemia), as previously mentioned, can be caused by low albumin, as well as renal failure. It can also be caused by massive blood transfusions. This is because something called citrate is added to stored blood to prevent it from clotting. Calcium in the body binds to the citrate, causing it to go lower.

Patients with hypocalcemia often will have no symptoms at all. However, if it gets low enough, you may see EKG changes, seizures, muscle weakness or irritability, and bronchospasm. Muscle irritability includes tetany (muscle spasms). You can check for this by assessing your patient for Chvostek's or Trousseau's sign. Chvostek's sign is when the facial muscles contract after tapping on the facial nerve. Trousseau's sign is when the muscles in the hand and forearm spasm after the brachial artery is occluded for 3 minutes (Usually accomplished by inflating a blood pressure cuff higher than the systolic pressure.

Patients with hypercalcemia may feel tired or weak. If it gets high enough, it can also lead to confusion and eventually coma. Other symptoms include increased urination (polyuria), kidney stones, constipation, nausea, ulcers, and arrhythmias.

Carbon Monoxide (CO, Carboxyhemoglobin)

- **Purpose**: Determine Carbon Monoxide Poisoning

- **Mnemonic**: "The O2 Sat won't slide with Carbon Monoxide"

- **Normal**: < 3% (or < 12% for smokers)

You've heard the horror stories about entire families falling asleep and never waking up because of carbon monoxide poisoning. I'm sure you've seen the many carbon monoxide detectors available in stores right next to the smoke detectors. It's a scary thing because you never know when you are being exposed to it until you start getting symptoms. It has no color, taste, or smell. If a patient comes in, it will be difficult to pick up on right away because it doesn't affect the pulse oximetry reading. They might be showing 100%, but they are actually hypoxic. This is because pulse oximetry measures oxygenated blood, not differentiating between Oxygen (O2) and Carbon Monoxide (CO).

If your patient is found to have CO poisoning, the treatment is fairly simple: give them oxygen. Give them lots of oxygen. This will help get rid of the CO in the blood and replace it with O_2. Common causes of CO poisoning include smoke, gas stoves, gas heaters, and car exhaust.

Carcinoembryonic Antigen (CEA)

- **Purpose**: Help diagnose and treat certain cancers

- **Mnemonic**: "CEA: Cancer Elevates Also"

- **Normal**: < 2.5 ng/mL (< 5 ng/mL for smokers)

- **Increased**: Chron's Disease, Cirrhosis, Certain Cancers, Peptic Ulcers, Inflammatory Conditions

CEA is a type of molecule that is produced normally during the embryo stage of human development. It is produced in the GI tract, but only in tiny amounts after we're born. Because of this, the levels are normally very low. If the levels are increased, then there is something going on that isn't normal. This test is most commonly used to help diagnose certain cancers (often for GI type cancers) and to help aid in the treatment. CEA is usually high in cases of cancer, but will begin to fall after successful treatment. If a tumor is removed, but the numbers stay high, then it may mean that there is still something there. Very high levels can indicate that cancer has metastasized.

The problem with this test is that it can also be elevated when there is a benign tumor. It might also be higher in smokers, patients with liver disorders, inflammatory bowel, or pancreatitis. This is why a high CEA level doesn't necessarily mean that there is cancer. It is simply used as an aid, along with all of the other tools we have at our disposal.

CD4 Count (T-Helper Cells)

- **Purpose**: 1. Determine Progression of HIV (Risk for Infection), 2. Diagnose Leukemia

- **Mnemonic**: "To see what AIDS has in store, check the CD4"

- **Normal**: 600 – 1500 cells/µL

- **Increased**: Leukemia, Lymphoma
- **Decreased**: Immunodeficiency Diseases (HIV/AIDS), Patients who've received organ transplants

CD4 cells, also known as T-Helper Cells, are instrumental in helping the body fight off infection. HIV stands for Human Immunodeficiency Virus, a name which tells us that our immune system is not up to par when this disease takes hold. In fact, it causes the body to attack itself. As HIV progresses, the CD4 count gets lower and lower without treatment. This will eventually lead to AIDS when the count gets very low (below 200).

As the CD4 count drops, it increases the risk for infection. Infections and complications from AIDS are what eventually lead to death. CD4 counts, in combination with other labs, help in keeping track of HIV's progression and guide treatment.

CD4 counts can also be used to diagnose Acute Myelocytic Leukemia (AML) and differentiate between other types of leukemias.

Chloride (Cl)

- **Purpose**: Electrolytes

- **Mnemonic**:
  - ➢ "Cation = (+) Positive"
  - ➢ "Anion = (-) Negative"

- **Normal**: 98 – 106 mEq/L

- **Increased**: Respiratory Alkalosis, Dehydration, Cushing Syndrome, Hyperparathyroidism, Multiple Myeloma, Anemia, Eclampsia, Metabolic Acidosis, Kidney Problems, Hyperventilation
- **Decreased**: Fluid overload, CHF, SIADH, Excessive Vomiting, Respiratory Acidosis, Addison Disease, Hypokalemia, Burns, Metabolic Alkalosis, Diuretics

This is a very common test that you'll often see with other labs in the BMP (basic metabolic panel) and CMP (comprehensive metabolic panel). This is not the time for a huge lecture on fluids and electrolytes, so let's just review the basics. Electrolytes have either a positive charge (cation) or a negative charge (anion). They react with each other to maintain a balance inside of the body. Chloride is an anion which keeps the balance with sodium (a cation). Chloride is not very original, so it plays copycat and does whatever sodium does. If sodium is lost in the urine, sure enough, chloride is there to follow. If sodium decides to build up in the body, chloride will be right next to it.

Chloride levels are used in conjunction with other tests to find out what's going on with a patient. For example, it can indicate if the patient is dehydrated. Remember that sodium will rise during dehydration, and chloride will follow suit. But it can also help diagnose acidosis or alkalosis by acting as a buffer. When a patient becomes acidotic, the hydrogen (H) levels will increase. When this happens, it forces bicarb (HCO3) to move out into the extracellular space, which is where chloride likes to hang out. To maintain balance, some chloride will shift back into the cell.

In a nutshell, you can't really tell much of anything with just a chloride level. But when you have a plethora of other labs at your disposal, you can begin to get a clearer picture of your patient's condition. Now you also don't have to wonder anymore why one of the most common fluids you'll hang is Sodium Chloride.

Coombs Test

- **Purpose**: Cross-matching blood, prenatal testing

- **Mnemonic**: "Coombs 'Combs' for antibodies in blood"

- **Normal**: Negative

The Coombs test can be either "direct" or "indirect." The direct test is done to see if a patient has autoimmune hemolytic anemia. This is when the body basically attacks itself, specifically by destroying the red blood cells. The indirect Coombs test is used for a couple of different reasons. The first is for pregnant women to find out if they have any problems with their blood that could end up causing hemolytic disease in the baby. The most widely used reason for the indirect test is to match up patient and donor blood prior to transfusion.

As I'm sure you're aware, all blood has to be tested and matched before transfusing. If the wrong blood type is given, the results could be catastrophic, ranging from a slight fever to death. During cross-matching, it is important to determine not only the blood type, but also for antibodies which may cause a reaction. This is where the indirect Coombs test comes in. It enables the lab to find out if antibodies are present before the blood is given to a patient.

Creatine Kinase (CK, CPK, Creatine Phosphokinase)

- **Purpose**: Determine muscle damage

- **Mnemonic**: "If the muscle is at play, then check the CK"

- **Normal**:
  - 55 – 170 units/L (Male)
  - 30 – 135 units/L (Female)

- **Increased**: Anything affecting the muscles of the heart, skeleton, or brain

This test is used to find out if there has been any muscle damage, and if so, to what extent. It is most commonly used to check for injury to the heart muscle, but can also check for skeletal muscle or neurological injuries. If your patient has a heart problem such as an MI (myocardial infarction, "heart attack"), the CK will rise, but will return to normal in 2-3 days unless the damage continues.

There are 3 specific isoenzymes that show where the muscle damage happened. If the damage is myocardial in nature, the CK-MB isoenzyme will be higher. If it is skeletal, the CK-MM will be higher. Lastly, if the muscle damage is neurological (and sometimes pulmonary), the CK-BB will be elevated. The enzyme levels can help indicate not only the level of damage that occurred, but also when the damage occurred.

CK-MB: MI, Myocarditis, arrhythmias, cardiac arrest

CK-MM: Muscular dystrophy, surgery, seizures, shock, trauma, low potassium, rhabdomyolysis

CK-BB: Pulmonary embolism (PE), central nervous system problems, adenocarcinoma

Creatinine (Cr)

- **Purpose**: Evaluate kidney function

- **Mnemonic**: "High Cr = Crappy Renal function"

- **Normal**: 0.5 – 1.2 mg/dL

- **Increased**: Renal Disease, UTI, Dehydration, Nephropathy, Rhabdomyolysis,   Acromegaly
- **Decreased**: Decreased Muscle Mass

Creatinine is a test used primarily to see how the kidneys are functioning. It is released by skeletal muscle and is eliminated solely by the kidneys. This is also the case with the BUN, which is often used in conjunction with the creatinine. With renal damage, the kidneys are unable to clear these substances, so their levels rise. This can happen acutely (rhabdomyolysis, dehydration, acute tubular necrosis) or chronically (renal cancer, kidney failure). If the kidney function is severely impaired, it can lead to very serious problems and dialysis may be needed.

Creatinine Clearance (CC, eGFR)

- **Purpose**: Evaluate Kidney Function

- **Mnemonic**:
  - ➤ "High GFR = Good Function Renally"
  - ➤ "If there's low clearance, check the kidney's appearance"

- **Normal**:
  - ➤ 107 – 139 mL/min (male)
  - ➤ 87 – 107 mL/min (female)
  - ➤ Values decrease with age
  - ➤ eGFR: >60 mL/min/1.73m2

- **Increased**: Pregnancy, Increased Cardiac Output, Exercise
- **Decreased**: Kidney Disease, Liver Disease, Dehydration, CHF, Shock

After creatinine is released by skeletal muscle, it is eliminated by the kidneys. Creatinine clearance is a measure of how well this substance is being eliminated, and is a way to gauge the GFR (glomerular filtration rate). Therefore, the higher the number, the more efficient the kidneys are performing. As we get older, the GFR and creatinine clearance decreases mostly due to decreased muscle mass.

A 24-hour urine test is necessary to obtain the creatinine clearance level. However, the GFR can be estimated using blood tests and patient information. Levels may be increased after exercise and pregnancy. They will likely be decreased when kidney function is impaired.

Cytomegalovirus (CMV)

- **Purpose**: Determine type of infection

- **Mnemonic**: "CMV = Common Mono-like Virus"

- **Normal**: Negative

CMV is a type of virus that is most often contracted before birth or as a young child, but can occur at any time. You can contract such infections through body fluids and blood transfusions. Unfortunately, there is no cure and can come and go as it pleases. Usually, it stays inactive unless your immune system is compromised. It is not uncommon for there to be no symptoms. If there are symptoms, it can often mimic mononucleosis. You might see fever, stomach ulcers, diarrhea, seizures, blindness, pneumonia, or hepatitis. In very extreme cases, encephalitis and even coma may happen.

D-Dimer

- **Purpose**: Diagnosing DIC, Risk for clots

- **Mnemonic**: "D-Dimer = Diagnose DIC"

- **Normal**: < 250 ng/mL

- **Increased**: DIC, Surgery, Fibrinolysis, DVT, PE, Sickle Cell Anemia

The D-Dimer test is a good indicator of risk level for blood clots, and therefore embolic events (PE, Stroke, MI). It measures plasmin and thrombin activity. When these are high, there is a greater chance of the blood clotting. It is also tested to check for the effectiveness of anticoagulant therapy.

D-Dimer is often used in the diagnosis of DIC (Disseminated Intravascular Coagulation). This is a condition that happens for various reasons, but is where the clotting activity becomes out of control. At first, this can lead to embolic events and lack of blood supply to vital organs. Later as the clotting proteins are overused and consumed, it becomes very difficult for the body to stop bleeding. DIC is a very serious complication that can quickly lead to death if not diagnosed and treated quickly. The D-Dimer can help diagnose this, along with other tests.

Erythrocyte Sedimentation Rate (Sed Rate)

- **Purpose**: Determine inflammation

- **Mnemonic**: "Check the sed rate to confirm an inflammatory state"

- **Normal**:
  - Up to 15 mm/hr (Men)
  - Up to 20 mm/hr (Women)

- **Increased**: Renal Disease, Inflammatory Conditions, Certain Anemias, Infection
- **Decreased**: Sickle Cell Anemia, Polycythemia Vera, Certain Meds

The sed rate is usually ordered to determine if there is inflammation going on in the body, and to what extent. What it is really measuring is the rate at which RBCs sediment (settle) in a solution over time. Unfortunately, it is very non-specific, so it will not diagnose anything for you. However, it can point you in the right direction. For instance, if you think the patient has an inflammatory autoimmune disorder, such as rheumatoid arthritis, an increased sed rate would tell you that your head is in the right place.

Sedimentation rate may be increased with certain medication, pregnancy, renal failure, malignant cancers, anemia, infection, and of course, inflammatory diseases. You might see a decreased level in polycythemia vera or sickle cell disease, or with certain medications.

Factor V Leiden

- **Purpose**: Determine presence of this Factor V disorder

- **Mnemonic**: "If there's a problem with Factor V (Five), then the clotting is in overdrive"

- **Normal**: Negative

Factor V is one of the proteins in the body that plays an important role in the coagulation process. Factor V Leiden is what you get when there is a defect in the gene. The blood becomes more prone to clotting, creating a greater risk of DVT.

In the coagulation cascade, protein C normally helps to decrease the amount of clotting. But in Factor V Leiden, it isn't able to do this because of the defect. In the US, it is the most prevalent blood coagulation disorder that is inherited.

The Factor V Leiden mutation can be either heterozygous (two different alleles of the gene) or homozygous (2 of the same alleles). Patients with heterozygous Factor V Leiden have a small increased risk for clots, while those with the homozygous form have a much higher risk.

Follicle-stimulating Hormone (FSH)

- **Purpose**: Determine reproductive system problems

- **Mnemonic**: "FSH = Freaking Sex Helper"

- **Normal**:
  - Male: 1.42 – 15.4 IU/L
  - Female: 1.37 – 9.9 IU/L   (Follicular Phase)
  - Female: 6.17 – 17.2 IU/L   (Ovulatory Peak)
  - Female: 1.09 – 9.2 IU/L   (Luteal Phase)
  - Female: 19.3 – 100.6 IU/L (Postmenopause)

- **Increased**: Menopause, Pituitary Tumor, Castration, Polycystic Ovaries, Puberty, Testicular Damage
- **Decreased**: Malnutrition, Stress, Pituitary Failure, Pregnancy

FSH is a hormone that is released by the anterior pituitary gland, which is attached to the brain. It is an important part of the reproductive system that plays many different roles in men and women. Testing the FSH levels can help find more information about fertility problems, menopause, ovarian cysts, and issues with the testicles.

A high FSH level can indicate that menopause has started, a pituitary tumor is present, there is damage to the testicles, or puberty is about to start (in adolescents). A low FSH level may be due to recent weight loss, pregnancy, or under-producing of eggs. The Luteinizing Hormone (LH) is often used as a guide along with the FSH to help diagnose and evaluate some of these issues.

Glucose

- **Purpose**: Determine blood sugar levels

- **Mnemonic**:
  - ➤ "Good Livers Unselfishly Convert Our Sugar Everyday"
  - ➤ "Beta cells secrete Insulin = BI = Brings It Down"
  - ➤ "Alpha cells secrete Glucagon = AG = Adds Glucose"

- **Normal**: 70 – 110 mg/dL

- **Increased**: Diabetes, Stress, Cushing Syndrome, Renal Disease, Diuretics, Pancreatitis, Steroids, Acromegaly, High Sugar Diet
- **Decreased**: Insulin Administration, Malnutrition, Hypothyroidism, Addison Disease, Liver Disease, Hypopituitarism

This is a test most of you are probably somewhat familiar with. It is one of the most common labs to be drawn, and can be done so at bedside or even by patients in their own homes. There are a plethora of over-the-counter options for glucose testing machines, as well as the supplies to do it. To obtain the test, you simply have to clean the area with alcohol, prick the area with a lancet, and place a drop of blood onto the testing strip. Of course, the test can also be obtained in a blood sample that is sent to the lab. It will come up as a part of the BMP (Basic Metabolic Panel) or CMP (Comprehensive Metabolic Panel).

The liver can produce glucose as needed, as well as store it for later if it's not needed. When you eat something, any glucose from it is utilized by the body for various functions. Often, we eat too much sugar, so it either needs to be stored for later or eliminated from the bloodstream somehow. The liver converts the glucose to glycogen and stores it for later. Glucose can also be decreased by insulin.

Insulin is secreted from the beta cells of the pancreas from the Islets of Langerhans (remember this...it's a common test question). When glucose is high (hyperglycemia), insulin is released to get the extra glucose to the liver and to the rest of the tissues.

What happens when glucose levels are too low (hypoglycemia)? Another substance, known as glucagon, is secreted from the alpha cells of the pancreas from the Islet of Langerhans. Glucagon tells the liver that the sugar is low and something needs to be done. In response, the liver converts the stored glycogen into glucose and releases it.

Islet of Langerhans (pancreas)

Insulin: beta cells

Glucagon: alpha cells

In diabetic patients, there is some part of this communication that is messed up. In type I diabetes, the problem is that there is no insulin, or not enough insulin, being produced from the pancreas. In type 2 diabetes, the problem is that the body becomes resistant to the insulin that is being secreted. In both cases, glucose rises if there is no treatment.

Hyperglycemia: If glucose gets too high too quickly, it can lead to a condition known as Diabetic Ketoacidosis (DKA – usually in type I) or Hyperglycemic Hyperosmolar Nonketotic Coma (HHNK – usually in type II). If it isn't taken care of, it can cause the patient to go into a coma or cardiac arrest. There are also many long-term effects related to diabetes. If a patient doesn't keep their glucose levels under control, it can eventually lead to very serious problems, such as cardiac disease, nerve damage, and kidney disease. The nerve damage can lead to neuropathies (numbness, tingling, pain), often in the hands or feet, due to abnormal nerve sensation. Patients can even experience this in the eyes (retinal neuropathy), causing vision problems and even blindness.

Hypoglycemia: If glucose gets too low, it can cause a patient to become lightheaded, confused, shaky, diaphoretic (sweaty). They might get palpitations, blurred vision, or slurred speech. If left without treatment, it can eventually lead to coma or even death.

Glucose-6-phosphate Dehydrogenase (G6PD) Screen

- **Purpose**: Determine G6PD Deficiency

- **Mnemonic**: "Lack of G6PeeDee = destruction of RBeeCee"

- **Normal**: Negative

G6PD is an enzyme that aids in the function of red blood cells. When a patient doesn't have enough of this enzyme, the red blood cells may start to get destroyed (hemolysis). It is a condition which is always present, but doesn't cause problems unless there is a trigger. Once the trigger is removed, the body will soon return to normal and working red blood cells will be reproduced. It is an X-linked trait, meaning that men are more likely to have it. Women who have the deficiency often have no symptoms.

Common Triggers:
Infection
Stress
Many Drugs (including aspirin, NSAIDS, and sulfa meds)
Certain Foods (especially fava beans)

Glycated Hemoglobin (HbA1c)

- **Purpose**: Tests long-term diabetes control

- **Mnemonic**: HbA1(one)c = High Blood sugars Are Out of Control

- **Normal**: < 6%

- **Increased**: Poorly Controlled Diabetes, Pregnancy, Post-Splenectomy
- **Decreased**: Renal Disease, Hemolytic Anemia, Prolonged Blood Loss

This test is most commonly used to see how well patients have controlled their diabetes over a long-term period of time (about 3-4 months). HbA1c is a component of hemoglobin that combines with glucose stronger than any other component. An RBC has a life-span of around 4 months, which is why this test is able to tell what the glucose levels have been in that timeframe. If the level is greater than 6-7%, it can indicate that treatment is not effective or that the patient has not been keeping their sugars under control.

Growth Hormone (GH, HGH)

- **Purpose**: Diagnose Growth Disorders

- **Mnemonic**: "GH = Get Huge"

- **Normal**:
  - < 5ng/mL (Men)
  - < 10 ng/mL (Women)

- **Increased**: Exercise, Acromegaly, Diabetes, Anorexia, Stress, Hypoglycemia, Surgery
- **Decreased**: Dwarfism, GH Deficiency, Hyperglycemia, Pituitary Insufficiency, Failure to Thrive

Growth Hormone is a gift that is secreted by the anterior pituitary gland. Its function does exactly what you think it does—it helps us grow. It has many other functions also, but this is the primary thing it does until the end of puberty. Sometimes, the anterior pituitary doesn't secrete enough GH, which may cause growth deficiencies and even dwarfism. If too much is secreted, you might get gigantism or acromegaly.

You may have heard of athletes getting in trouble for taking HGH, which stands for Human Growth Hormone. This is basically a synthetic version of natural Growth Hormone. Taking this allows the athletes to get bigger, more muscular, and stronger. It has also been offered as a supplement to the general public and has been claimed to be beneficial to overall health.

Hematocrit (Hct)

- **Purpose**: Determine need for blood transfusion

- **Mnemonic**:
  - ➤ "Low Hematocrit can be due to Hemorrhage"
  - ➤ "If the bleeding won't quit and they're pressure is s#it, check the hematocrit"

- **Normal**:
  - ➤ 38-50% (Men)
  - ➤ 35-45% (Women)

- **Increased**: Burns, Dehydration, Polycythemia Vera, Eclampsia, COPD, Heart Disease
- **Decreased**: Anemia, Lymphoma, Renal Disease, Liver Disease, Hyperthyroidism, Hemorrhage, Pregnancy, Multiple Myeloma, Rheumatoid Arthritis, Leukemia, Prosthetic Heart Valves

Hematocrit is one of the most common lab values requested and can be found as part of the CBC (Complete Blood Count). It measures how much the red blood cells (RBCs) are a part of the total blood volume and is shown as a percentage. The hematocrit rises or falls with the hemoglobin and is usually around 3 times its value. For example, if the hemoglobin is 10, the hematocrit is probably around 30. Both of these labs are used as a guide for blood transfusion requirements. When the HCT is decreased, the patient has anemia, which can be caused by various reasons. If the HCT is increased, it can mean that the patient has one of several possible problems, including dehydration, erythrocytosis, or polycythemia vera.

Hemoglobin (Hgb)

- **Purpose**: Determine need for blood transfusion

- **Mnemonic**: "Hemorrhage will lead to low Hemoglobin"

- **Normal**:
  - 13.5-17.5 g/dL (men)
  - 12-15.5 g/dL (women)

- **Increased**: Dehydration, Heart Disease, Polycythemia Vera, COPD, Burns
- **Decreased**: Anemia, Hemorrhage, Splenomegaly (enlarged spleen), Kidney Disease, Lymphoma, Lupus, Malnutrition, Sarcoidosis

Hemoglobin is a very common lab and will show up as part of the CBC (Complete Blood Count). It is a type of protein, present in the red blood cells (RBCs), that functions to carry oxygen throughout the body. This often goes hand-in-hand with the hematocrit, and is usually in a 1:3 ratio. For example, if the hemoglobin is 10, then the hematocrit is probably around 30. Both values rise and fall together. A low hemoglobin indicates that the patient has anemia, a condition that can be caused by many things, such as hemorrhage or certain diseases. If the hemoglobin is high, it could also be due to a number of possibilities, including dehydration or polycythemia vera. The hemoglobin value is commonly used as a guide for the need of blood transfusions.

High-Density Lipoproteins (HDL)

- **Purpose**: Evaluate cholesterol levels

- **Mnemonic**:
  - ➤ "HDL = Helpful cholesterol"
  - ➤ "Keep HDL High"
  - ➤ "Keep LDL Low"

- **Normal**:
  - ➤ 40-50 mg/dL (Men)
  - ➤ 50-59 mg/dL (Women)

- **Increased**: Exercise, Genetics
- **Decreased**: Low Protein, Genetics, Metabolic Syndrome, Liver Disease

HDL is part of the lipid profile, and provides insight into the cholesterol level in the body. While LDL (Low-Density Lipoproteins) is considered bad, HDL is commonly known as the "good" cholesterol. This is because it is responsible for carrying harmful things from your body, such as fat, triglycerides, and even the LDLs, to the liver. The liver then breaks them down and gets those bad things out of your body via bile. The higher the HDL is, the better. The lower the LDL is, the better.

HDL is evaluated by itself, as well as with the LDL and total cholesterol. These lab values can help monitor for cholesterol treatment and identify risk for heart disease, stroke, and lung problems.

Human Chorionic Gonadotropin (hCG, β-hCG)

- **Purpose**: Determine Pregnancy

- **Mnemonic**: "HCG: Human Coming, Girl!"

- **Normal**: < 5.0 mU/mL

- **Increased**: Pregnancy, Certain Cancers

The hCG is a common blood test used to confirm pregnancy. It can also be used to diagnose a miscarriage, diagnose an ectopic pregnancy, and find out how far along the pregnancy is. It is often tested to make sure a woman isn't pregnant before surgery, X-rays, or anything that has the potential to harm a baby. When used in conjunction with other tests, hCG can help diagnose abnormalities with the baby, such as Down syndrome.

The test can either be qualitative or quantitative. A qualitative test simply tells you if there is hCG present above normal values. This is measured from the urine and what causes the "+" symbol to appear in a home pregnancy test. A quantitative hCG measures the specific amount in the blood (β-hCG).

International Normalized Ratio (INR)

- **Purpose**: Evaluate anticoagulant therapy, determine risk for bleeding

- **Mnemonic**: "Coumad<u>IN</u> <u>R</u>aises the INR"

- **Normal**:
  - ➢ < 1.0
  - ➢ 2.0-3.0 (therapeutic)
  - ➢ 2.5-3.5 (very high risk for clots)

- **Increased**: Coumadin, Liver Disease, Vitamin K Deficiency, DIC, Massive Blood Transfusions

INR is a value that is derived from the Prothrombin Time (PT). It is used primarily to measure the effectiveness of warfarin (Coumadin), but is also used to check for bleeding risk (especially in a patient with liver problems). Coumadin is an anticoagulant taken by patients who are at a high risk for blood clots (atrial fibrillation, DVT history, artificial heart valves, etc). These patients are kept at a therapeutic range, as you don't want the INR to be too high or too low. The higher the INR, the thinner the blood, and the greater the risk is for bleeding. The lower the INR, the thicker the blood, and the greater the risk is for clotting. Patients who are on Coumadin must go in regularly to ensure that this number is kept within range.

If the INR gets too high, there are a few ways to bring it down. The first thing you will need to do is stop taking the Coumadin. You can give IV vitamin K, which is a sort of antidote to Coumadin. In a pinch, FFP (fresh frozen plasma) can be given to bring it down quickly, though it's not a long-term solution.

Patients who have liver disease, DIC, or clotting factor disorders may have an increased INR also. This is due to the disruption of the coagulation cascade, which is a conversation suited for another day.

Lactate Dehydrogenase (LDH)

- **Purpose**: Detect generalized tissue damage or infection

- **Mnemonic**: "LDH: Liberated when Damaged, then High (levels)"

- **Normal**: 105-333 IU/L

- **Increased**: MI, Generalized Disease or Injury, Liver Disease, Kidney Disease, Pulmonary
                 Disorders, Certain Cancers, Pancreatitis

LDH is a substance that is in the cells of most of the tissues in the body. When these cells are damaged, the LDH is released into the bloodstream, causing an increase in the lab value. The problem is that it is very hard to pinpoint where the damage is because it can be found in so many places. There are isoenzymes of LDH that can give a better clue of the location source, but these labs aren't drawn very often.

LDH may rise in certain types of anemia, infection, kidney or liver disease, broken bones, some cancers, and muscle injuries. Sometimes this lab is drawn in cerebrospinal fluid (CSF) to differentiate between bacterial and viral meningitis (high LDH usually points to bacterial). It may also be tested from pleural, peritoneal, and pericardial fluid to help diagnose certain problems, such as liver cirrhosis and CHF.

Lactic Acid (Lactate)

- **Purpose**: Determine level of tissue hypoxia

- **Mnemonic**: "Think they're sep*tic*? Check the lac*tic* (acid)"

- **Normal**:
  - 5 – 20 mg/dL (venous sample)
  - 3 – 7 mg/dL (arterial sample)

- **Increased**: Sepsis, Carbon Monoxide Poisoning, Diabetes, Liver Disease, Genetics

The 2 main types of metabolism are aerobic and anaerobic. The body likes to function on aerobic metabolism, in which there is plenty of oxygen available for the tissues. In this state, glucose gets metabolized to CO_2 and H_2O. Anaerobic metabolism happens when the amount of oxygen to the tissues decreases. Glucose then gets metabolized to lactic acid, rather than CO_2. As the lactate increases more and more, patients can develop lactic acidosis. This is something that can happen in septic shock, severe liver disease, carbon monoxide poisoning, diabetes, and with certain medications (such as metformin).

Lecithin/Sphingomyelin Ratio (L/S Ratio)

- **Purpose**: Determine fetal lung maturity

- **Mnemonic**:
  - "High L/S = Happy Lung Status"
  - "Low L/S = Lousy Lung Status"

- **Normal**: > 2.0

- **Increased**: Better Lung Development
- **Decreased**: Inadequate Lung Development

The L/S Ratio is used to test how well the lungs of a fetus have matured. The sample is taken from the amniotic fluid, a process called an amniocentesis. Surfactant is a very important substance that allows the lungs to work properly, but is even more vital for premature babies. Lecithin (L) and Sphingomyelin (S) are a big part of the make-up of surfactant.

The L/S ratio helps to determine the risks and benefits of delivering a baby prematurely. The higher the ratio, the better, but 2.0 is usually a good number to shoot for. If the ratio is lower than 1.5, then there is a much higher risk of the baby having difficulty breathing after birth. Certain medications, such as betamethasone (a

steroid), can be used to help increase the
surfactant production.

Lipase

- **Purpose**: Identify pancreas problems

- **Mnemonic**: "Amylase and Lipase tells you about the Pancreas(e)"

- **Normal**: 0 – 160 units/L

- **Increased**: Pancreas Disorders, Renal Disease, Peptic Ulcers, Bowel Obstruction, Duct   Obstructions

The pancreas secretes lipase, which takes triglycerides and turns them into fatty acids. If the cells in the pancreas are damaged, lipase levels begin to increase in the blood. The lipase is usually drawn along with the amylase, as they both often move in the same direction. Persistent problems, such as pancreatitis or pancreatic cancer, will cause these levels to remain high.

Although an increased level of lipase will usually show signs of pancreatic problems, there are other things that could cause it as well. For example, high levels can also be seen with kidney failure, bowel obstruction, peptic ulcers, and with certain medications.

Low-density Lipoproteins (LDL)

- **Purpose**: Evaluate cholesterol levels

- **Mnemonic**:
  - ➢ "LDL = Lousy cholesterol"
  - ➢ "Keep HDL High"
  - ➢ "Keep LDL Low"

- **Normal**: < 130 mg/dL

- **Increased**: Genetics, Poor Diet, Nephrotic Syndrome, Hypothyroidism, Liver Disease, Multiple Myeloma, Cushing Syndrome
- **Decreased**: Genetics, Hyperthyroidism, Malnutrition

LDL is part of the lipid profile, and provides insight into the cholesterol level in the body. While HDL is commonly known as the "good" cholesterol, LDL (Low-Density Lipoproteins) is considered bad. This is because LDLs carry cholesterol into the blood vessels, while HDLs help get rid of cholesterol and other harmful things. Having cholesterol in your blood vessels is not awesome. This cholesterol can build up over time, causing atherosclerosis, narrowing the blood vessels more and more each day. This increases the risk of clots and thrombotic events.

LDL is evaluated by itself, as well as with the HDL and total cholesterol. These lab values can help monitor for cholesterol treatment and identify risk for heart disease, stroke, and lung problems. The higher the HDL is, the better. The lower the LDL is, the better.

Luteinizing Hormone (LH)

- **Purpose**: Determine reproductive system problems

- **Mnemonic**: "LH: Love Hormone"

- **Normal**:
  - Male: 1.24 – 7.8 IU/L
  - Female: 1.68 – 15 IU/L   (Follicular Phase)
  - Female: 21.9 – 56.6 IU/L (Ovulatory Peak)
  - Female: 0.61 – 16.3 IU/L (Luteal Phase)
  - Female: 14.2 – 52.3 IU/L (Postmenopause)

- **Increased**: Menopause, Pituitary Tumor, Castration, Polycystic Ovaries, Puberty, Testicular Damage
- **Decreased**: Malnutrition, Stress, Pituitary Failure, Pregnancy

LH is a hormone that is released by the anterior pituitary gland, which is attached to the brain. It is an important part of the reproductive system that plays many different roles in men and women. Testing the LH levels can help find more information about fertility problems, menopause, ovarian cysts, and issues with the testicles.

A high LH level can indicate that menopause has started, a pituitary tumor is present, there is damage to the testicles, or puberty is about to start (in adolescents). A low LH level may be due to recent weight loss, pregnancy, or under-producing of eggs. The Follicle-stimulating Hormone (FSH) is often used as a guide along with the LH to help diagnose and evaluate some of these issues.

Lyme Disease

- **Purpose**: Detect presence of Lyme Disease

- **Mnemonic**: "Lyme Disease is transmitted by Leeching Deer ticks"

- **Normal**: Negative

Contrary to popular belief, you don't get Lyme disease from eating rotten limes. All jokes aside, there are certain types of ticks (especially deer ticks) that carry bacteria called Borrelia burgdorferi. This bacteria is the cause of eventual Lyme disease. Other ways of getting the disease may be possible, but extremely unlikely. Ticks usually have to be attached to some part of the body for at least 1-2 days before transmission can happen.

After being infected, the first sign is usually a skin lesion with a rash-like appearance at the site of the bite. Later, you might get a fever, sore muscles, enlarged lymph nodes, headache, and generalized weakness. If Lyme disease persists, you might see rashes in other areas, severe joint swelling and pain, palpitations, nerve pain, brain/spinal cord inflammation, memory issues, or Bell's Palsy (facial droop).

When testing for Lyme disease, it is usually done in two phases. First, the EIA (enzyme immunoassay) is drawn. If the EIA test is negative, then there is no Lyme disease. If it is positive or unclear, then the second phase is done, which requires doing the Western Blot test. If the Western Blot shows positive, then you have Lyme disease.

Magnesium (Mg)

- **Purpose**: Check electrolytes

- **Mnemonic**: "If you see torsades, the mag might be at odds"

- **Normal**: 1.5 – 2.1 mEq/L

- **Increased**: Renal Disease, Hypothyroidism, Diabetes, Addison Disease, High intake of Antacids containing magnesium
- **Decreased**: DKA, Malnutrition, Renal Disease, Liver Disease, Hypoparathyroidism

Magnesium is an important electrolyte, but is not part of the BMP (Basic Metabolic Panel) or the CMP (Comprehensive Metabolic Panel). It has many functions, most importantly keeping the heart happy. It is mostly located on the inside of the cells in the body. In the bone is where you'll find half of all magnesium.

High magnesium might be caused by kidney problems, diabetes, hypothyroidism, and Addison disease. One of the most common reasons is due to taking antacids that contain magnesium. Hypermagnesemia symptoms can range from nausea and vomiting to weakness to slurred speech.

Low magnesium can happen when patients aren't getting enough nutrition, during acidosis, and in chronic renal disease. You might also see it in alcoholics, hypoparathyroidism, and lack of absorption of magnesium. Hypomagnesemia may cause arrhythmias, weakness, confusion, and seizures.

Low magnesium is a common cause of a lethal arrhythmia called torsades de pointes, which means "twisting of the points." It is a type of ventricular tachycardia that appears to be twisting at the QRS complex. This is why you'll see magnesium as a standard part of code carts.

Parathyroid Hormone (PTH, Parathormone)

- **Purpose**: Regulate Calcium and Phosphate

- **Mnemonic**: "PTH regulates CAP: Calcium And Phosphate"

- **Normal**: (Intact) 10 – 65 pg/mL

- **Increased**: Hyperparathyroidism, Certain Cancers, Rickets, Renal Disease, Hypocalcemia, Vitamin D Deficiency
- **Decreased**: Hypomagnesemia, Graves Disease, Sarcoidosis, Hypercalcemia, Hypoparathyroidism, Excessive Vitamin D Intake

When the calcium level in the body is low, the parathyroid gland responds by releasing PTH into the bloodstream. It stimulates the osteoclasts in the bone to release calcium and causes the kidneys to reabsorb it, as well as increase the absorption by the GI system. PTH also helps to regulate the phosphate levels by various methods.

PTH might be high if the patient has hyperparathyroidism, low calcium, vitamin D deficiency, and in ectopic tumors that cause PTH production. PTH might be low if the patient has hypoparathyroidism, high calcium, and parathyroid surgery. When measuring the PTH, the calcium level needs to be measured as well so they can be compared.

Partial Thromboplastin Time (PTT)

- **Purpose**: Evaluate coagulation function

- **Mnemonic**: Coagulation Factors: "It costs $1 to $2 to get 5 beers between the hours of 8-12"

- **Normal**: 60 – 70 Seconds (aPTT 30 – 40 seconds)

- **Increased**: Clotting Disorders, Heparin, Vitamin K Deficiency, Liver Disease, DIC
- **Decreased**: Certain Cancers, Early in DIC

The PTT is one of several ways to determine how well a patient is coagulating, or how well an anticoagulant is working. In the coagulation cascade, PTT tells us about the intrinsic pathway, as well as the common pathway. It tests the function of many coagulation factors, including I, II, V, VIII, IX, X, XI, and XII. A common medication used for anticoagulation is Heparin. PTT is often used to monitor its effectiveness, especially if it is being used as a continuous drip. Heparin has a very quick effect, with the PTT changing within hours after titrating an IV drip.

Another version of the PTT is the activated partial thromboplastin time (aPTT). In the lab, an "activator" is added to the blood sample, which helps to make the clotting time faster. This makes the range for a normal result narrower.

PTT results may be increased when certain drugs are given, such as heparin. You might also see it if patients have a problem with one of the clotting factors, liver problems, DIC, or deficiency of Vitamin K. It could be decreased in certain types of cancer, as well as in DIC during the first phases of the disorder.

Phosphate (PO4)

- **Purpose**: Check Electrolytes

- **Mnemonic**: "PTH helps to regulate PHosphaTe"

- **Normal**: 3.0 – 4.5 mg/dL

- **Increased**: Renal Disease, Anemia, Lymphoma, Acidosis, Acromegaly, Hypoparathyroidism, Hypocalcemia, Sarcoidosis, Liver Disease
- **Decreased**: Chronic Antacid intake, Hyperparathyroidism, Sepsis, Alkalosis, Rickets, Malnutrition, Hypercalcemia, Vitamin D Deficiency, DKA

Phosphate is often the "forgotten electrolyte" since it is rarely, if ever, critical information. There is organic and inorganic phosphate. Organic phosphate is how it mostly exists in the body, as a part of other compounds. Inorganic phosphate is a much smaller portion of the total phosphate, but is the one that we are testing for. You can find it on the inside of the cells (intracellular). It likes to hang out in the bones with calcium, but some of it floats around in the blood. Phosphate is regulated by metabolism of ingested foods, the parathyroid hormone (PTH), and of course by the kidneys.

If a patient has hypophosphatemia (low phosphate), it might be because of taking antacids long-term, hyperparathyroidism, sepsis, malnutrition, hypercalcemia, alcoholism, Vitamin D deficiency, or diabetic ketoacidosis (DKA). Most patients won't have any symptoms, but you may see weakness, confusion, or complaints of bone pain.

If a patient has hyperphosphatemia (high phosphate), it could be due to renal failure, anemia, cancer, acidosis, liver problems, hypoparathyroidism, hypocalcemia, or rhabdomyolysis. Most patients won't have any symptoms, but you may see nausea and vomiting, anorexia, trouble breathing, fatigue, and trouble sleeping.

Platelets (Thrombocytes)

- **Purpose**: Evaluate risk for bleeding

- **Mnemonic**:
  - ➢ "Low Platelets may aid in Bloodletting"
  - ➢ "High Thrombocytes help create a thrombus"

- **Normal**: 150,000 – 400,000/mm3

- **Increased**: Polycythemia Vera, Rheumatoid Arthritis, Anemia (iron-deficient), After Splenectomy, Malignancy
- **Decreased**: Hypersplenism, Infection, Certain Anemias, Lupus, DIC, Hemorrhage, Leukemia, Chemotherapy

The platelet count is a very important part of the CBC (complete blood count). It tells you how well the blood is clotting. The higher the platelets, the better the clotting. The lower the number, the more difficult it is to clot (therefore increasing the bleeding risk). A patient is usually said to have thrombocytopenia when the platelet count goes below 100,000. Numbers this low might cause you to pause before surgeries and certain procedures, since the bleeding risk is higher. A critical number would be below 50,000, and below 20,000 might cause spontaneous bleeding without being provoked.

When the platelet level is high, it is called thrombocytosis. This is not usually as much of a concern as with thrombocytopenia, but should be noted. It might be caused by a number of things, including malignancy, rheumatoid arthritis, anemia, and polycythemia vera.

Thrombocytopenia is a major concern, as the risk for bleeding goes up more and more as the platelet count falls. It could be caused by several problems, such as infection, chemotherapy, hemorrhage, leukemia, DIC, lupus, anemia, and thrombocytopenia disorders.

Potassium (K)

- **Purpose**: Check Electrolytes

- **Mnemonic**: "K= EKG Changes (Electrolyte Kills Good Cardiac)"
                (Yes, I know it's not grammatically correct, but it works!)

- **Normal**: 3.5 – 5.0 mEq/L

- **Increased**: Diet, Renal Disease, Certain Diuretics, Infection, Dehydration, Acidosis, Hemolysis
- **Decreased**: Burns, Diet, Excessive Vomiting and Diarrhea, Surgery, Trauma, Cystic Fibrosis, Certain Diuretics, Cushing Syndrome, Insulin, Glucose

Potassium is one of the most important electrolytes in the body. It plays a vital role in many functions, especially in the cardiac system. It is the main cation (positive charge) inside of the cells. But the major effects it has are due to the concentration of potassium extracellularly (in the serum).

The kidneys have a major part in excreting potassium, but don't have much to do with making sure it stays in the body if needed. Most of the potassium is obtained in our food and drinks. If you don't get enough from there, the level can drop quickly. This is why many patients have to take potassium supplements on a daily basis.

In patients with kidney problems, the potassium can't be cleared from the body as it should, so the levels begin to rise. In patients with renal failure on dialysis, the potassium can get out of control between treatments. You can also see hyperkalemia with acidosis, major burns, dehydration, infection, hypoaldosteronism, and too much intake (via the diet or IV).

As previously mentioned, hypokalemia can happen because of lack of intake through the diet. It may also be due to excessive vomiting, diarrhea, cystic fibrosis, ascites, hyperaldosteronism, Cushing syndrome, and certain medication administration (insulin, glucose, calcium, diuretics).

A cardinal sign of hyperkalemia is a peaked T wave (higher than usual) on the EKG tracing. You can also see arrhythmias, a widened QRS segment and the ST segment might be depressed. Patients may feel irritable, nauseous, or have diarrhea.

Hypokalemia may present with cardiac issues also, such as arrhythmias, flat T waves, and large U waves (not always noticeable on a normal EKG). Patients may also develop an ileus (lack of movement in the intestine, often causing a blockage) with a low potassium. Weakness may develop in these patients, and possibly feelings of paralysis at very low levels.

Prostate-specific Antigen (PSA)

- **Purpose**: Screen for Prostate Cancer

- **Mnemonic**: "PSA: Prostate Screen After 50"

- **Normal**: 0 – 2.5 ng/mL

- **Increased**: Prostate Cancer, BPH, Prostatitis

PSA is a substance found in all men, located primarily in the lumen of the prostate. However, this substance can be detected at much higher numbers in the bloodstream when there is a problem with the prostate, especially cancer. This test is most commonly used to screen for prostate cancer. The higher the PSA, it typically means the higher the probability of cancer and the bigger the tumor might be.

PSA levels may also be slightly increased in other non-cancerous problems, such as BPH (Benign Prostatic Hypertrophy). This is a condition where the prostate is enlarged, often causing discomfort, such as pain or difficulty urinating. But it is benign, meaning non-cancerous and usually not dangerous.

It is recommended that men above 50 get tested once a year or once every 2 years, depending on the initial PSA level. If patients have a high risk of getting prostate cancer, they should get a PSA screening by age 40. Note that these recommendations are not definitive, and some believe that men don't need to be screened until 75 if they aren't high risk.

Prothrombin Time (PT)

- **Purpose**: Evaluate anticoagulant therapy, determine risk for bleeding

- **Mnemonic**: "High PT: Hemorrhage risk from Prolonged bleeding Time"

- **Normal**: 11.0 – 12.5 seconds

- **Increased**: Coumadin, Liver Disease, Vitamin K Deficiency, DIC, Massive Blood Transfusions

The PT is a lab value that is used to assess how well the body is clotting, and therefore the risk of bleeding. The INR (International Normalized Ratio) is derived from the PT, so these lab values are usually evaluated together. It gauges the effectiveness of the extrinsic and the common pathways of the coagulation cascade. The specific factors include I, II, V, VII, and X. The longer the PT is, the greater the risk of bleeding is (or the greater the anticoagulant therapy is working).

Patients who are at risk for blood clots must be placed on anticoagulant therapy. One of the most common medications these patients take is Coumadin. This increases the PT and INR, but the INR is what is usually referred to when assessing these patients. Other things that may cause the PT to be increased include liver problems,

Vitamin K deficiency, factor disorders, DIC, and massive blood transfusion.

If the PT/INR gets too high, there are a few ways to bring it down. The first thing you will need to do is have the patient stop taking the Coumadin. You can give IV vitamin K, which is a sort of antidote to Coumadin. In a pinch, FFP (fresh frozen plasma) can be given to bring it down quickly, though it's not a long-term solution.

Rapid Strep Test (RADT)

- **Purpose**: Diagnose strep throat

- **Mnemonic**: "Rapid Strep Test: Rule out Strep Throat"

- **Normal**: Negative

This is a test that can be used quickly, determining if a patient has the bacteria that causes strep throat within 10-20 minutes. The bacteria in question is Streptococcus pyogenes (group A streptococcus). A throat culture can also be done, but this takes much longer to get results. Since the rapid test is so accurate, the culture is rarely ordered unless something other than strep throat is suspected.

Signs of strep throat are the same types of symptoms you would see with most bacterial infections. This includes fever, headache, nausea, dehydration, and body aches. There will obviously be a sore throat, along with redness and inflammation. It's common to see blood or white/yellow spots on the tonsils or in the back of the throat. If strep throat is not treated properly, it may lead to rheumatic fever (This is a common test question). This is a very dangerous condition that can cause several problems, including severe damage to the heart.

Red Blood Cells (RBC)

- **Purpose**: Evaluate for anemia

- **Mnemonic**: "RBC: Red Bone marrow Creation"

- **Normal**:
  - ➤ 4.7 – 6.1 million cells/µL (Male)
  - ➤ 4.2 – 5.4 million cells/µL (Female)

- **Increased**: Polycythemia Vera, COPD, Heart Disease, Dehydration, Pulmonary Fibrosis
- **Decreased**: Hemorrhage, Anemia, Prosthetic Heart Valves, Pregnancy, Volume Overload, Renal Disease, Certain Cancers, Hemolysis

The RBC is drawn as a part of the CBC (Complete Blood Count). It measures the amount of red blood cells per 1 mm^3 that are in venous blood. They are produced in the bone marrow and contain hemoglobin molecules that transport oxygen and carbon dioxide throughout the body. When there are no problems present, a red blood cell can typically survive for 120 days. Rarely is the RBC count looked at on its own. It is usually compared and evaluated with the hemoglobin, hematocrit, and platelet count.

The RBC count might by higher than usual if the patient has pulmonary fibrosis, cor pulmonale, dehydration, polycythemia vera, and congenital heart disease. It can also be seen in places that are high in altitude. The RBC count is often low in anemia, hemorrhage, pregnancy, endocarditis, some cancers, bone marrow problems, chemotherapy, renal problems, and rheumatoid arthritis.

Rheumatoid Factor (RF)

- **Purpose**: Diagnose Rheumatoid Arthritis

- **Mnemonic**: "RF = Rigid, Firm joints"

- **Normal**: Negative

Rheumatoid factor is most often used to diagnose and evaluate rheumatoid arthritis. It can also be used to rule out rheumatoid arthritis, opening the door for the possibility of other inflammatory diseases. The test is not a guaranteed diagnosis. Just as there can be false-positives, a negative result doesn't necessarily mean that rheumatoid arthritis isn't present.

Rheumatoid arthritis is an autoimmune disorder where the body basically starts attacking itself. It causes a great deal of inflammation and affects mostly the joints, causing intense pain for many patients. Although the joints are the primary areas affected, the disease can cause many other problems. For example, it can also affect the heart, kidneys, lungs, skin, blood vessels, etc.

Other possible reasons for an increased rheumatoid factor include lupus, Sjogren syndrome, and other autoimmune diseases. You can also see it in patients with liver or kidney problems, leukemia, syphilis, tuberculosis, and endocarditis.

Schilling Test

- **Purpose**: Determine cause of B12 deficiency, diagnose pernicious anemia

- **Mnemonic**: "Don't be a Schill, take a B12 pill"

- **Normal**: 8-40% excreted in urine in 24 hours

- **Decreased**: Pernicious Anemia, Scleroderma, Liver Disease, Malabsorption, Lymphoma, Hypothyroidism, Chron's Disease

The Schilling test is to find out if vitamin B_{12} is being absorbed the way that it should. Absorption usually happens in the ileum of the intestine after combining with intrinsic factor. If any of the B12 isn't needed, it gets sent out of the body in the urine. If there is a problem absorbing the B12, something called pernicious anemia can develop. This happens because B12 is needed to make red blood cells (RBCs). If there's not enough, anemia will occur. The intrinsic factor helps the B12 get absorbed, so a lack of it can also cause a problem.

To administer the test, first radioactive vitamin B12 is given by mouth and injected into muscle. In the first 24 hours, the urine will show at least

8-10% of the B12 that was administered. If it is normal, great! If it is abnormal, the next step is to repeat the test, adding intrinsic factor this time. If this 2nd part of the test is normal, then the patient likely has pernicious anemia. If it is abnormal also, then it is probably a lack of intrinsic factor. This can be caused by a number of things, including liver disease and tapeworms.

The Schilling test is not used often today, as many practitioners are relying more on other diagnostic information to determine B12 deficiency.

Sickle Cell Screening (Hemoglobin S)

- **Purpose**: Diagnose Sickle Cell disease/trait

- **Mnemonic**: "Sickle cell can hurt like hell"

- **Normal**: Negative

The sickle cell screen is ordered for patients who are at high risk of having the disease or trait. It is a genetic problem in which the RBCs (red blood cells) become misshapen into a crescent like form instead of its usual round form. This is caused by the presence of Hgb S, rather than the typical Hgb A. If the patient is homozygous (both alleles are the same) for Hgb S, then they have sickle cell disease. If the patient is heterozygous (2 different alleles) for Hgb S, then they have the trait for the disease (but not the disease itself).

The crescent shape that the RBCs form resemble a sickled shape, hence the name of the disease. In this shape, it becomes difficult for the cells to pass through the capillaries. They begin to get plugged and start to build up.

This can lead to very severe pain throughout the body when there is a sickle cell "crisis." It may also cause generalized fatigue, infections, problems with vision, and slow growth. These patients also have a shorter life expectancy.

Sodium (Na)

- **Purpose**: Check Electrolytes

- **Mnemonic**:
  - ➤ "Sodium = Same Osmolality" So...
  - ➤ "High Sodium = High Osmolality"
  - ➤ "Low Sodium = Low Osmolality"

- **Normal**: 135 – 145 mEq/L

- **Increased**: High Intake, Cushing Syndrome, Diabetes Insipidus, Sweating, Hyperaldosteronism
- **Decreased**: Low Intake, Addison Disease, Edema, Pleural Effusion, CHF, Diarrhea, Vomiting, Excessive Water Ingestion, SIADH, Renal Disease, Ascites

The sodium level is one of the most common labs drawn and is part of the BMP (basic metabolic panel) and CMP (comprehensive metabolic panel). It is the most abundant cation (+ charge) outside of the cells in the blood.

There are many things that play a role in the regulation of sodium, with the kidneys being the major determining factor. The renin-angiotensin-aldosterone system helps the body retain sodium when the levels are low and get rid of sodium when the levels are high. It is also controlled by the things people eat in their diets.

Unfortunately, all of these systems can fail or simply can't keep up.

When low sodium (hyponatremia) occurs, patients may feel tired or weak, restless, and confused. They might also feel nauseous, have muscle spasms, and a headache. If it gets really low, it could eventually lead to seizures and even coma.

A lot of the same symptoms may arise when high sodium (hypernatremia) occurs, including weakness, fatigue, and restlessness. It can also cause seizures and coma if it gets high enough. Two cardinal signs of high sodium are excessive thirst and edema (generalized swelling).

Another thing to think about is the osmolality in your body. This is a way to measure how concentrated the fluid is in your blood, as well as your urine. If you are dehydrated, your osmolality is high. If you have too much fluid, your osmolality is low.

Imagine a glass of salt water sitting in the sun. As the water evaporates, the ratio of salt to water will begin to increase. The more water that is lost to evaporation, the greater the osmolality becomes of the contents in the glass. More salt plus less water equals a higher osmolality. This is easy to translate back to the body, especially since the two main substances we're dealing with are salt (Na) and water ($H2O$).

High Na + *Low* H2O = *High* Concentration = *High* Osmolality

Low Na + *High* H2O = *Low* Concentration = *Low* Osmolality

Thromboelastography (TEG)

- **Purpose**: Assess coagulation quality

- **Mnemonic**: "TEG: Thrombocyte Evaluation Grade"

- **Normal**:
  - K Value: 1 – 4 min
  - α-Angle: 47 – 74°
  - R Value: 4 – 8 min
  - MA: 55 – 73 mm

The TEG is a fairly new test that is used to measure the quality of coagulation in the body. There are several tests that can evaluate the risk of bleeding, such as the PT, PTT, INR, and platelet count. Platelets (thrombocytes) are an important part of clotting. The higher the number of platelets you have, the easier it is to clot. But that doesn't tell the whole story.

Not all platelets are created equally, as some work better than others. Two patients may have identical labs with a platelet count of 100,000, but one will be at a higher risk of bleeding. This is where the TEG comes in. It tells not only how many platelets there are, but also how efficient those platelets are working.

The TEG measures how fast clotting occurs (K Value, α-Angle), the reaction time (R Value), and the strength of the clot (G-value, MA-Maximum Amplitude). This can all be put together to form the Coagulation Index (CI), an overview of the TEG.

This test is ordered when it is vital to know how much of a bleeding risk a patient is, particularly if their platelet count is borderline. It is not commonly done, but can be useful for high risk surgery and other procedures.

Thyroid-stimulating Hormone (TSH)

- **Purpose**: Diagnose thyroid problems

- **Mnemonic**: "TSH = This is Secreted more in Hypothyroidism"

- **Normal**: 2 – 10 mU/L

- **Decreased**: Hyperthyroidism, Graves Disease

- **Increased**: Hypothyroidism, Hashimoto's Thyroiditis

The TSH is used in conjunction with other lab values to help evaluate thyroid function and diagnose thyroid disorders. TSH is released from the pituitary, after being stimulated by TRH (Thyroid Releasing Hormone). TSH does exactly what its name says—it stimulates the thyroid hormones. When T3 (triiodothyronine) and T4 (thyroxine) get low, TSH springs into action to get them motivated again.

When a patient has hypothyroidism (decreased function), there is a decrease in T3 and T4. This causes the TSH to rise in an attempt to bring these levels up. Therefore, a high TSH would indicate the possibility of primary hypothyroidism.

However, it is sometimes the case that TSH secretion is being blocked by something, such as a tumor or trauma. This is secondary hypothyroidism. In this scenario, the TSH levels would be low, along with the T3 and T4 levels.

Once a patient is diagnosed with hypothyroidism, the TSH can still be used to monitor how well the treatment is working. When patients are given thyroid replacement medication, a TSH level that continues to be high might indicate that the dose needs to be increased.

In patients with hyperthyroidism, you would find the TSH levels to be low, while at the same time, the T3 and T4 levels would be high.

Thyroxine (T4)

- **Purpose**: Diagnose thyroid problems

- **Mnemonic**:
  - ➤ "Free T4: Functioning T4"
  - ➤ "Total T4: Tied-up T4"

- **Normal**:
  - ➤ Total: 4 – 12 mcg/dL
  - ➤ Free: 0.8 – 2.8 ng/dL

- **Increased**: Graves Disease, Hepatitis, Pregnancy, Thyroiditis, Hyperthyroidism, Thyroid   Adenoma
- **Decreased**: Cretinism, Cirrhosis, Pituitary Insufficiency, Myxedema, Cushing Syndrome, Renal Disease, Deficient Iodine

T4 is used in conjunction with other lab values to help evaluate thyroid function and diagnose thyroid disorders. The thyroid gland secretes T4(thyroxine) and T3 (Triiodothyronine). It is called T4 because it contains 4 atoms of iodine. TSH (Thyroid-stimulating Hormone) is released from the pituitary, after being stimulated by TRH (Thyroid-releasing Hormone). TSH does exactly what its name says—it stimulates the thyroid hormones (T3 and T4).

T4 is much more abundant than T3, but it isn't as strong. Almost all of the T4 in the body is attached to proteins, such as albumin. A very small amount is unattached, free to roam its surroundings on its own. The protein-bound T4 isn't meaningless, but the free T4 is the only form that is metabolically active.

The total T4 level includes both forms, while the free T4 level only counts the active form. If there are any changes in protein levels, the total T4 will also be different. For example, a patient with low albumin will have a low total T4 but a normal free T4. Because of this, free T4 is a better measure of thyroid functioning.

Total Cholesterol

- **Purpose**: Evaluate cholesterol levels

- **Mnemonic**: "Total Cholesterol: Sum of the good (HDL), bad (LDL), and the ugly (Triglycerides)"

- **Normal**: Less than 200 mg/dL

- **Increased**: Poor Diet, Genetics, Hyperlipidemia, Hypothyroidism, Pregnancy, Stress, Hypertension, Diabetes, MI
- **Decreased**: Genetics, Malnutrition, Hyperthyroidism, MI, Liver Disease, Certain Anemias, Stress, Sepsis

The total cholesterol is used, along with several other labs, to evaluate cholesterol levels. It is a measure of sum of the HDL, LDL, and a portion of the triglycerides. Cholesterol can build up over time, causing atherosclerosis, narrowing the blood vessels more and more each day. This increases the risk of clots and thrombotic events.

While total cholesterol is important to know, it doesn't tell the entire story. Each portion of this lab value must be assessed individually as well. When the total cholesterol is a little high, it could be because the HDL is too high. In this case, it's not a bad thing, since it is better when HDL is high. However, the total value could be high because the LDL is too high. This would suck, since LDL is considered the "bad" cholesterol.

Total Protein

- **Purpose**: Determine nutritional status

- **Mnemonic**: "TAG: Total = Albumin + Globulin"

- **Normal**: 6.4 – 8.3 g/dL

Total protein is an indicator of the overall nutritional status of a patient. Albumin, along with globulin, makes up most of the total protein in the body. Sometimes, total protein is referred to when determining if a patient's albumin is low.

Albumin is the largest component of the total protein in the blood. It is produced in the liver and its job is to maintain the colloidal osmotic pressure. This pressure makes sure that fluid is balanced between the tissues in the body and the capillaries. Normally, it is inclined to pull water into the capillaries. When there is a problem, water can leak out into the tissue, causing edema.

Some examples of problems causing low albumin include malnutrition, liver disease, and severe burns. It is also common to have a decreased albumin in late pregnancy. If your patient's albumin is low, it can be replaced via IV. But the underlying cause will need to be addressed, or it will keep dropping. Albumin may be increased when a patient is dehydrated. However, dehydration is typically a fairly easy thing to diagnose, so an albumin level is not normally needed in this case.

Triglycerides

- **Purpose**: Evaluate cholesterol levels

- **Mnemonic**: "If the food is fried, it will raise your triglyceride(s)"

- **Normal**: Less than 150 mg/dL

- **Increased**: Hyperlipidemia, Pregnancy, MI, Diabetes, Hypertension, Hypothyroidism, Glycogen Storage Disease, Poor Diet, Genetics
- **Decreased**: Genetics, Malnutrition, Hyperthyroidism

Triglycerides are measured, along with other labs, to determine a patient's cholesterol level and risk for other problems. They are a form of fat made in the liver and like to tag along with lipoproteins (LDLs and VLDLs). The main function of triglycerides is to store energy, but end up getting dumped into fatty tissues when there is too much of it.

Patients with high triglycerides, as with other cholesterol levels, are at a much higher risk for heart disease. They are also more prone to thrombotic events, such as stroke, pulmonary embolism, or heart attack.

Triiodothyronine (T3)

- **Purpose**: Diagnose thyroid problems

- **Mnemonic**: "T3 is less than T4, but longer (triiodothyronine) is stronger (than Thyroxine)"

- **Normal**: 100 – 200 ng/dL

- **Increased**: Graves Disease, Hepatitis, Pregnancy, Thyroid Adenoma, Thyroiditis, Hyperthyroidism
- **Decreased**: Hypothyroidism, Liver Disease, Cushing Syndrome, Cretinism, Myxedema, Malnutrition, Pituitary Insufficiency, Insufficient Iodine, Renal Disease

T3 is used in conjunction with other lab values to help evaluate thyroid function and diagnose thyroid disorders. The thyroid gland secretes T4 (thyroxine) and T3 (Triiodothyronine). It is called T3 because it contains 3 atoms of iodine. TSH (Thyroid-stimulating Hormone) is released from the pituitary, after being stimulated by TRH (Thyroid-releasing Hormone). TSH does exactly what its name says—it stimulates the thyroid hormones (T3 and T4).

T4 is much more abundant than T3, but it isn't as strong. Almost all of the T3 in the body is attached to proteins, such as albumin. A very small amount is unattached, free to roam its surroundings on its own. The protein-bound T3 isn't meaningless, but the free T3 is the only form that is metabolically active.

Usually, the lab value you will see is the total T3. Because of the attachment to proteins, a low albumin level will cause the T3 level to be low also. The same holds true if the albumin is high.

Troponin

- **Purpose**: Diagnose MI (heart attack)

- **Mnemonic**: "If the heart is moanin', check the troponin"

- **Normal**:
  - ➢ Troponin I: Less than 0.03 ng/mL
  - ➢ Troponin T: Less than 0.1 ng/mL

- **Increased**: MI, any Myocardial Injury

The troponin level is drawn in patients who are suspected of having some kind of cardiac event, though usually helps to evaluate a myocardial infarction (heart attack). Troponins hang out in skeletal and cardiac muscle, but can be zoned in on specific areas. The area we are usually concerned with is cardiac muscle. The cardiac troponins that are drawn are troponin T and troponin I. Most labs will usually just give the value of one or the other, but they both tell the same information.

When a patient has a heart attack, these troponins are released into the bloodstream and can be detected within 2-3 hours, and will continue to rise as long as injury is still occurring. Once a troponin is found to be elevated, doctors will usually order serial labs drawn to check the extent of injury and know when it has stopped. When the troponin gets to its highest level, it is said to have "peaked" before it begins its decent back down to normal. It can stay high for up to 2 weeks after an attack.

Although this lab is usually drawn to evaluate an infarction, elevated levels can mean many other things. This might include CHF (congestive heart failure), pulmonary embolism, unstable angina, cardiac trauma, renal failure, hypertension, and arrhythmias.

Urine Culture and Sensitivity (C&S)

- **Purpose**: Diagnose UTI and identify cause

- **Mnemonic**: "Urine C & S: Corrupted Stream"

- **Normal**: Less than 10,000 bacteria/mL of urine
  (More than 100,000 indicate UTI)

- **Increased**: Urinary Tract Infection

In this test, a urinary tract infection (UTI) can be diagnosed. The type of bacteria or yeast that is causing the UTI can also be identified so the appropriate treatment may be used. The urinary tract consists of the kidneys, bladder, ureters, and urethra. Typically though, the culprit is the bladder.

This test should be done before any antibiotics are started, since they can disrupt the results. Once a UTI is confirmed, antibiotics can be tested on the urine to see which one it is the most sensitive to. This will help in choosing the correct treatment.

A urine C&S is often done along with a urinalysis, which also will point to infection. The white blood count (WBC), pH, bacteria level will be elevated. Sometimes, a urine culture won't be done until after a positive urinalysis.

Ventilation/Perfusion Scan (V/Q Scan)

- **Purpose**: Diagnose pulmonary embolism (PE)

- **Mnemonic**: "To see if you perfuse, check your Q's"

- **Normal**: No pulmonary embolism (normal perfusion)

The V/Q scan is a measure of the ventilation (V) and perfusion (Q) ratio to determine the likelihood of a pulmonary embolism (PE) being present. The V in ventilation is easy to remember, but the Q for perfusion can be a little more difficult. See the mnemonic above.

A patient who has had a PE has experienced a blockage in the blood flow to the lungs. This will cause a disruption in the perfusion. The issue is that an abnormal V/Q scan can also mean several other problems with the lungs. This can include pneumonia, COPD, asthma, lung cancer, bronchitis, and tuberculosis.

Because this nuclear scan can show abnormal for many reasons, a PE isn't diagnosed this way as often as it once was. Instead, tests such as CT, MRI, ultrasound, pulmonary angiography, and other blood tests are frequently turned to. These, in combination with a patient's symptoms, can usually confirm with reasonable certainly whether or not a PE has occurred.

Very-low-density Lipoproteins (VLDL)

- **Purpose**: Evaluate Cholesterol Levels

- **Mnemonic**: "VLDL: Very Lousy Cholesterol"

- **Normal**: 7 – 32 mg/dL

- **Increased**: Genetics, Poor Diet, Nephrotic Syndrome, Hypothyroidism, Liver Disease, Multiple Myeloma, Cushing Syndrome
- **Decreased**: Genetics, Hyperthyroidism, Malnutrition

VLDLs are measured, along with other labs, to determine a patient's cholesterol level and risk for other problems. This is a lipoprotein that is often forgotten about, with HDL and LDL usually taking up most of the spotlight. However, it is something that shouldn't be taken lightly. VLDLs are the primary carriers of triglycerides, although LDLs also play a part in this.

In all honesty, VLDLs aren't as big of a concern, but they can still increase the risk for heart disease and vascular problems. Cholesterol can build up over time, causing atherosclerosis, narrowing the blood vessels more and more each day. This increases the risk of clots and thrombotic events.

VLDL is evaluated by itself, as well as with the LDL, HDL, and total cholesterol. These lab values can help monitor for cholesterol treatment and identify risk for heart disease, stroke, and lung problems. The higher the HDL is, the better. The lower the LDL and VLDL is, the better.

White Blood Cells (WBC, Leukocytes)

- **Purpose**: Determine presence and severity of infection

- **Mnemonic**: "If there's an infection to fight, check the blood count that's white"

- **Normal**: 5,000 – 10,000 /mm3

- **Increased**: Infection, Inflammation, Stress, Trauma
- **Decreased**: Autoimmune Disease, Bone Marrow Disorder, Certain Meds

The WBC count is very common and is drawn as part of the CBC (complete blood count). A high count (leukocytosis) most often means that there is an infection present somewhere in the body. The WBC count rises as a way of fighting off the infection. It is very non-specific, so you never know which part of the body is causing the problem. It can also mean there is inflammation or tissue injury/death somewhere. Sometimes, if trauma has occurred or some type of stress, the WBC count may also rise.

A low WBC count (leukopenia) can be caused by anything that suppresses the immune system. This might be chemotherapy, bone marrow disease, and autoimmune diseases, such as AIDS.

When the WBC levels are low, it puts the patient at a very high risk for getting an infection. This is because there aren't enough attackers to fight anything off.

If a "CBC with diff" is ordered, this means that the doctor also wants so see the differential count of the WBCs. This is a measure of each type of leukocyte that makes up the white blood cells. They include the granulocytes (neutrophils, eosinophils, and basophils) and the nongranulocytes (lymphocytes, monocytes, and histiocytes).

NCLEX-Style Practice Questions

Test your lab value knowledge with these 110 NCLEX-style practice questions. This section just shows the question and answer choices. Jot down your answers and check them in the next section, which shows the correct answers and the rationales. If you'd prefer to see them now, feel free to skip ahead to page 207. Good Luck!

1. The patient has had a cough with blood-tinged sputum for 3 weeks. During differential diagnosis, the nurse knows that which of the following tests may be ordered to help rule out tuberculosis?

   a. Carcinoembryonic Antigen (CEA)
   b. Acid-Fact Bacillus (AFB)
   c. Coombs Test
   d. Cytomegalovirus (CMV)

2. The nurse has been made aware of the patient's increased Activated Clotting Time (ACT). In which of the following scenarios would this be an expected finding? Choose all that apply.

   a. Heparin therapy
   b. Thrombosis
   c. Liver Disease
   d. Coumadin therapy
   e. Psoriasis
   f. Myocardial Infarction

3. The nurse knows that the Brain Natriuretic Peptide (BNP) is an important lab result to follow in a patient with congestive heart failure (CHF). Which area of the body is this substance released from?

    a. Ventricles of the heart
    b. Atria of the heart
    c. Left lower lobe of the lungs
    d. Right middle lobe of the lungs

4. The student nurse is taking care of an 83-year-old male on hemodialysis. Which of the following statements indicates the need for further teaching?

    a. It is common for the creatinine to be *increased* in patients with kidney disease
    b. Blood Urea Nitrogen (BUN) is commonly *increased* in patients with kidney disease
    c. Blood Urea Nitrogen (BUN) is commonly *decreased* in patients with kidney disease
    d. It is common for the potassium to be *increased* in patients with kidney disease

5. While reviewing lab values, the nurse knows it is more important to pay attention to the ionized calcium, since the total calcium can be affected by which of the following?

    a. Bilirubin
    b. Ammonia
    c. Albumin
    d. Erythrocytes

6. You tap on your patient's facial nerve in an attempt to elicit a contraction response of the facial muscles. When the patient asks what you are doing, the most appropriate response would be which of the following?

    a. I am checking for Chvostek's sign to see if you may have a *high* calcium level
    b. I am checking for Chvostek's sign to see if you may have a *low* calcium level
    c. I am checking for Trousseau's sign to see if you may have a *high* calcium level
    d. I am checking for Trousseau's sign to see if you may have a *low* calcium level

7. A 53-year-old male patient was admitted
   24 hours ago with a myocardial infarction.
   The nurse is aware that which of the
   following lab results is most likely
   elevated?

   a. Glucose
   b. BUN
   c. INR
   d. CK-MB

8. Your patient with stage III kidney disease
   has been prescribed IV antibiotics. Which
   of the following lab values would be most
   helpful in identifying the glomerular
   filtration rate (GFR) and overall kidney
   function?

   a. Prothrombin time
   b. Creatinine clearance
   c. BUN
   d. Sodium level

9. The patient's lab results show an increased creatinine level. When the preceptor asks what it means, what would be the most appropriate response by the student nurse?

   a. It is usually indicative of kidney disease
   b. It suggests a problem with myocardial function
   c. It is usually indicative of liver disease
   d. It often means that there is a problem with the pancreas

10. The patient you are caring for has an elevated LDL level. In which of the following conditions would this lab result be most expected?

   a. Hypertension
   b. Hyperlipidemia
   c. Diabetes
   d. Hypothyroidism

11. The nurse knows that increased total cholesterol can lead to atherosclerosis, which increases the risk for which of the following?

    a. Pleural effusion
    b. Congestive Heart Failure
    c. Liver cirrhosis
    d. Myocardial infarction

12. The attending physician has ordered a ventilation/perfusion (V/Q) scan after your patient suddenly started complaining of chest pain and shortness of breath. This test is often performed to rule out which of the following conditions?

    a. Myocardial infarction
    b. Hepatitis
    c. Appendicitis
    d. Pulmonary embolism

13. Your patient has been admitted for appendicitis, and currently has a fever and tachycardia. Which of the following lab results would you most likely expect in this scenario?

    a. Increased white blood cell (WBC) count
    b. Increased red blood cell (RBC) count
    c. Increased prothrombin time (PT)
    d. Decreased prothrombin time (PT)

14. Secretion of Atrial Natriuretic Peptide (ANP) would most likely be stimulated in which of the following conditions?

    a. Congestive Heart Failure
    b. Hyponatremia
    c. Dehydration
    d. Hypotension

15. 10 units of regular insulin has been ordered for your patient with type 2 diabetes. Under normal circumstances, which part of the body is insulin secreted from?

   a. Alpha cells of the pancreas
   b. Anterior pituitary gland
   c. Beta cells of the pancreas
   d. Posterior pituitary

16. A patient who was admitted with Lyme disease is concerned about transmitting the disease to his family. You assure him that it is not a contagious disease and is usually transmitted by which of the following?

   a. Deer
   b. Deer ticks
   c. Horse ticks
   d. Fleas

17. Your patient's lab results show an increased parathyroid hormone (PTH) level. Which of the following conditions may be the cause for this value? Select all that apply.

    a. Hyperparathyroidism
    b. Hypocalcemia
    c. Vitamin D deficiency
    d. Rickets
    e. Hypomagnesemia
    f. Hypercalcemia

18. Sickle cell disease is caused by the presence of which of the following?

    a. Hemoglobin A
    b. Hematocrit A
    c. Hemoglobin S
    d. Hemoglobin F

19. You are caring for a patient with B12 deficiency. Which of the following tests is helpful in determining the cause?

    a. Coombs test
    b. Chvostek's sign
    c. Schilling test
    d. Trousseau's sign

20. A patient who is being tested for thyroid disease is waiting to review the lab results with the physician. In regards to thyroxine (T4) and triiodothyronine (T3), which of the following statements are true?

    a. T3 is more abundant than T4
    b. T3 is weaker than T4
    c. T4 is more abundant than T3
    d. T3 and T4 are equal in abundance

21. While drawing an ABG, the nurse knows that which lab value will most likely cause acidosis?

a. Low PaCO2
b. High HCO3
c. High PaO2
d. High PaCO2

22. Your patient has just arrived back to the unit from the operating room. Initial lab results show a low hemoglobin and hematocrit. The patient is awake, sitting up in bed. Which of the following is the most likely to be ordered to specifically treat this?

a. Blood products
b. Broad-spectrum antibiotics
c. Immediate Intubation
d. Fluid restriction

23. A 22-year-old female patient is in the emergency room for intractable nausea and vomiting. The attending physician has ordered an hCG level (human chorionic gonadotropin). The nurse knows that which of the following diagnoses are being ruled out?

    a. Infection
    b. Myocardial Infarction
    c. Pregnancy
    d. Pulmonary Embolism

24. A 33-year-old female who had surgery on her left ankle 2 days ago now has an increased anion gap. This particular lab value is most likely to indicate which of the following conditions?

    a. Alkalosis
    b. Acidosis
    c. Increased bicarbonate
    d. Decreased hydrogen ions

25. Your patient's lab results show a decreased albumin level. After being produced in the liver, what is the main function of albumin?

    a. Maintain the colloidal osmotic pressure
    b. Control blood pressure
    c. Maintain sodium balance
    d. Control the blood-brain barrier

26. Your patient's lab results reveal an elevated bilirubin level. In which condition is this most likely related to?

    a. Renal failure
    b. Hepatitis
    c. Pulmonary edema
    d. Colitis

27. As a nurse, it is important to know which labs will be included with each panel that is ordered. Which of the following lab panels would include the alanine aminotransferase (ALT, SGPT) level?

a. Complete blood count (CBC)
b. Basic metabolic panel (BMP)
c. Renal Panel
d. Comprehensive metabolic panel (CMP)

28. Your patient has been diagnosed with Syndrome of Inappropriate ADH Secretion (SIADH). In which part of the body does production of ADH occur?

a. Adrenal glands
b. Thyroid gland
c. Hypothalamus
d. Parathyroid gland

29. A patient you are caring for is in Hyperglycemic Hyperosmolar Nonketotic Coma (HHNK). Which of the following lab values would you most likely expect to see?

    a. Low glucose
    b. High creatinine
    c. Low creatinine
    d. High glucose

30. Which of the following scenarios is the most likely cause of an increased C-reactive protein (CRP)?

    a. An infected wound
    b. Parkinson's disease
    c. Alzheimer's disease
    d. A steroid injection

31. Your patient's erythrocyte sedimentation rate (ESR) is elevated. Which of the following is incorrect regarding this lab result?

    a. It is a very specific diagnostic tool
    b. It may be elevated during infection
    c. It is often elevated during inflammation
    d. It measures the rate at which RBCs settle in a solution over time

32. A 53-year-old female has arrived at the doctor's office to review her most recent lab results. Every result is close to the normal range, with the exception of the follicle-stimulating hormone (FSH), which is elevated. Which of the following conditions may cause an elevated FSH? Select all that apply.

    a. Malnutrition
    b. Pituitary tumor
    c. Menopause
    d. Polycystic ovaries
    e. Pregnancy

33. You notice that your patient's lab results include an increased sodium level. Which of the following symptoms would they most likely present in relation to hypernatremia?

    a. Excessive hunger
    b. Clear urine
    c. Fever
    d. Excessive thirst

34. You are caring for a 47-year old male with lung cancer, who has been receiving chemotherapy for the last 6 months. The most recent lab results show a decreased white blood cell count. This puts the patient at an increased risk for which of the following?

    a. Infection
    b. Blood loss
    c. Muscle loss
    d. Muscle cramps

35. In a patient who is suspected to have tuberculosis, which of the following statements is correct?

    a. An AFB smear is more sensitive than an AFB culture

    b. An AFB smear will yield results much faster than an AFB culture

    c. An AFB smear is a definitive diagnosis of tuberculosis

    d. The most common body fluid to be tested for an AFB smear is urine

36. You are caring for a patient who has been admitted for surgery related to a positive BRCA test. Which of the following surgeries would you most likely expect to be done?

    a. Craniotomy

    b. Mastectomy

    c. Splenectomy

    d. Vasectomy

37. You are caring for a patient who is being treated for deep vein thrombosis (DVT). Which of the following disorders would cause the greatest risk for blood clots?

    a. Heterozygous Factor V Leiden
    b. Thrombocytopenia
    c. Homozygous Factor V Leiden
    d. Liver cirrhosis

38. The patient was found unresponsive at home by a family member. The family member states that the power was off and a generator was running in the living room when he got there. The patient stopped breathing by the time the paramedics arrived, but the oxygen saturation was 100%. Which lab value would you expect to be increased when the patient gets to the hospital?

    a. Carbon Monoxide (CO)
    b. PaO2
    c. Hemoglobin
    d. Hematocrit

39. Your patient's lab results revealed an increased carcinoembryonic antigen (CEA) level. This is indicative of which of the following?

    a. It always means cancer is present
    b. It never means cancer is present
    c. It may be caused by more than just cancer
    d. It can only be caused by cancer

40. A morbidly obese patient is admitted to your unit. The lab results show an elevated D-Dimer level. This typically indicates that the patient has a greater chance of which of the following risks?

    a. Liver damage
    b. infection
    c. Diabetes
    d. Blood clots

41. Lactate Dehydrogenase (LDH) may be drawn to detect which of the following conditions?

   a. High cholesterol
   b. Specific tissue damage or infection
   c. Generalized tissue damage or infection
   d. Certain sexually-transmitted diseases

42. Which of the following tests would be the most sensitive when trying to confirm the diagnosis of tuberculosis?

   a. Blood culture
   b. AFB Culture
   c. AFB smear
   d. Rapid strep test

43. A 62-year-old male has arrived to the ER by ambulance, complaining of chest pain. The care team is concerned that the patient is having a myocardial infarction, and begin appropriate treatment measures. Which of the following lab values would most likely be elevated in this scenario?

   a. INR
   b. Glucose
   c. Troponin
   d. Creatinine

44. In which of the following conditions would you expect your patient's adrenocorticotropic hormone (ACTH) to be elevated?

   a. Long-term steroid use
   b. Secondary Adrenal insufficiency
   c. Addison disease
   d. Hypopituitarism

45. Growth hormone (GH) may be decreased in which of the following conditions? Select all that apply?

a. Acromegaly
b. During exercise
c. Dwarfism
d. Pituitary insufficiency
e. During stress
f. During surgery

46. Your 43-year-old male patient has been admitted with acute pancreatitis. Which of the following lab values would you expect to be increased because of this condition?

a. Lipase
b. Calcium
c. Triglycerides
d. Thyroxine

47. During a code, you notice the patient's rhythm appear to resemble ventricular tachycardia, but with a twisting quality. You suspect that it is torsades de pointes, knowing that this condition is likely caused by which lab value?

    a. High magnesium
    b. High calcium
    c. Low magnesium
    d. Low calcium

48. Thromboelastography (TEG) is a fairly new test that would most likely be used to determine which of the following?

    a. Platelet quality
    b. Hemoglobin quality
    c. Hemoglobin count
    d. Platelet count

49. A patient with a decreased Thyroid-stimulating hormone (TSH) level is most likely to have which of the following conditions?

    a. Hypothyroidism
    b. Graves disease
    c. Hashimoto's thyroiditis
    d. Addison's disease

50. The parathyroid hormone (PTH) is responsible for causing the release of which of the following electrolytes when stimulated?

    a. Potassium
    b. Sodium
    c. Magnesium
    d. Calcium

51. Your patient's body has difficulty absorbing B12. Which of the following disorders would this most likely be associated with?

    a. Iron-deficient anemia
    b. Pernicious anemia
    c. Thrombocytopenia
    d. Leukemia

52. Which of the following lab values is the most likely to be increased when there is new bone growth, such as after fracture or during adolescents?

a. Amylase
b. Aspartate aminotransferase (AST)
c. Alkaline phosphatase (ALP)
d. D-dimer

53. The patient in metabolic alkalosis would most likely have which results on the arterial blood gas (ABG)?

a. pH 7.61, PaCO2 25, HCO3 23
b. pH 7.40, PaCO2 40, HCO3 24
c. pH 7.58, PaCO2 37, HCO3 32
d. pH 7.29, PaCO2 37, HCO3 14

54. A newborn who was born 24 hours ago has developed a yellowish tint to their skin, known as jaundice. The nurse knows that the increase of which of the following lab values is the most likely cause?

a. Albumin
b. Bilirubin
c. Bicarbonate
d. Ferritin

55. A rapid strep-test is often used in healthcare settings to quickly rule out strep throat. Patients who test positive and are left untreated are at a higher risk for developing which of the following conditions?

a. Rheumatic fever
b. Alzheimer's disease
c. Thyroid cancer
d. Diabetes mellitus

56. Upon reviewing your patient's lab results, you notice that the sodium level is elevated. This is most likely present in which of the following conditions?

a. Excessive water intake
b. Low osmolality
c. Pleural effusion
d. Dehydration

57. Which of the following lab values would most likely be expected in a patient who is in disseminated Intravascular Coagulation (DIC)?

a. Decreased PT
b. Increased glucose
c. Increased D-dimer
d. Increased platelet count

58. Antidiuretic hormone (ADH, vasopressin) is a lab value that can be used most effectively to identify which of the following conditions?

a. Diabetes type 1
b. Diabetes Insipidus
c. Diabetes type 2
d. Diabetic ketoacidosis (DKA)

59. You are taking care of a 65-year-old female with COPD who has smoked a pack of cigarettes per day for 45 years. The arterial blood gas (ABG) shows a pH of 7.29, PaCO2 of 58, and HCO3 of 24. What is the most appropriate classification for these results?

    a. Respiratory Acidosis
    b. Respiratory Alkalosis
    c. Normal ABG
    d. Metabolic Acidosis

60. Your patient has a chronically low phosphate (PO4) level. Which of the following conditions is the most likely contributing factor to this?

    a. Chronic antacid intake
    b. Hypocalcemia
    c. Hypoparathyroidism
    d. Acromegaly

61. A 29-year-old female with non-Hodgkin's lymphoma is admitted for a port placement. She has been getting chemotherapy treatments for the past 2 weeks. Her most recent lab results show a very low platelet count, putting her most at risk for which of the following?

   a. Blood clots
   b. Excessive Bleeding
   c. Myocardial infarction
   d. Cerebrovascular accident

62. A patient who was admitted 3 hours ago on the medical-surgical floor is found to have an increased Blood Urea Nitrogen (BUN). What are the most common causes of this lab result? Select all that apply.

   a. Kidney Disease
   b. Hypervolemia
   c. Dehydration
   d. COPD
   e. Urinary tract obstruction
   f. Hemorrhagic shock

63. A 28-year-old female who is being seen in the office is concerned about her family history of cancer. Which of the following lab tests might be helpful in determining her likelihood of developing breast cancer?

   a. CNCR
   b. BRCA
   c. ACTH
   d. RISK

64. Your patient has a history of congestive heart failure (CHF), and has been admitted with shortness of breath. Which lab value would you most likely expect to find?

   a. Increased Alaline Transaminase (ALT, SGPT)
   b. Decreased Aspartate Transaminase (AST, SGOT)
   c. Decreased Brain Natriuretic Peptide (BNP)
   d. Increased Brain Natriuretic Peptide (BNP)

65. Your patient was diagnosed with Human Immunodeficiency Virus (HIV) 5 years ago. Which of the following lab results will indicate how much the disease has progressed since that time?

    a. CD4 Count
    b. Amylase
    c. BRCA
    d. Fibrinogen

66. You are caring for a patient who just had major abdominal surgery. The doctor has ordered for 2 units of packed red blood cells (PRBCs) to be given. What is one way the blood bank can determine if antibodies are present in the patient's blood sample before transfusing any products?

    a. Arterial blood gas (ABG)
    b. Blood culture
    c. Coombs test
    d. Hemoglobin A1C

67. Chloride is an electrolyte that is classified as an anion. The nurse knows that this means it has which of the following properties?

a. Positive charge
b. Negative charge
c. Neutral charge
d. No charge

68. A 29-year-old female, who is 39 weeks pregnant, has been admitted to the labor and delivery unit. When going through her history, she states that she was once told she has an increased risk for blood clots. Which of the following lab values would correlate with this description?

a. Increased PTT
b. Presence of Factor V Leiden
c. Thrombocytopenia
d. Iron-deficiency anemia

69. Under normal circumstances, red blood cells (RBCs) have a lifespan of how long?

    a. 4 months
    b. 4 weeks
    c. 4 years
    d. 4 hours

70. A patient with suspected carbon monoxide poisoning has just arrived via ambulance to the emergency room. She is stable and breathing, but very tired and confused. Which of the following treatment options would be the most helpful in this situation?

    a. Oxygen via non-rebreathing mask
    b. IV epinephrine
    c. Raising the head of the bed
    d. Pain medication

71. A 23-year-old female is 7 months pregnant and has been having some abdominal pain and cramping. The obstetrician would like to determine the fetus' Lecithin/Sphingomyelin ratio. Which body fluid would you expect to be tested?

   a. Fetal blood
   b. Mother's blood
   c. Mother's Urine
   d. Amniotic fluid

72. Which of the following lab values would you most likely expect to see on an arterial blood gas (ABG) in a patient who is in diabetic ketoacidosis (DKA)?

   a. Increased pH
   b. Decreased PaCO2
   c. Increased base excess (BE)
   d. Decreased HCO3

73. Your patient with type I diabetes begins to feel weak and tired, and appears pale and diaphoretic. Alteration in which of the following labs is the most likely cause of these symptoms?

    a. Hemoglobin
    b. White blood cells
    c. Potassium
    d. Glucose

74. A patient is being educated on Glucose-6-phosphate-dehydrogenase (G6PD) deficiency. Which of the following statements would indicate that further teaching is required?

    a. It is a genetic y-linked disorder
    b. It is a condition in which the red blood cells may become damaged
    c. It is commonly triggered by infection, stress, and certain drugs and foods
    d. Men are more likely to inherit the disorder

75. You have decided to test for Trousseau's sign in a patient with hypocalcemia. Which of the following methods would best demonstrate this?

a. Occlude the radial artery for 3 minutes
b. Tap on the patient's cheek
c. Occlude the brachial artery for 3 minutes
d. Tap on the patient's palm

76. In an environment of anaerobic metabolism, which lab value is the most likely to be increased?

a. PaO2
b. Phosphorus (PO4)
c. Lactic acid
d. Hemoglobin

77. Your diabetic patient has had a consistently high glucose since admission 2 days ago. He states that his blood sugar is usually under control. Which of the following lab tests would be the most helpful in determining how well his diabetes has been controlled over the past 6 months?

    a. Glucose-6-Phosphate-Dehydrogenase (G6PD)
    b. Glycated Hemoglobin (HbA1c)
    c. Factor V Leiden
    d. Arterial blood gas (ABG)

78. You are caring for a patient with severe malnutrition and failure to thrive. The lab results show a decreased total protein, which is comprised of which 2 substances?

    a. Albumin and globulin
    b. Albumin and sodium
    c. Bile and globulin
    d. Albumin and bile

79. A patient who is on chronic Coumadin (warfarin) therapy is likely to have an increase in INR. The INR is derived from which of the following lab values, which is also likely to be elevated?

a. Hemoglobin
b. Platelets
c. Hematocrit
d. Prothrombin time

80. When a patient has a myocardial infarction, how soon can the increased troponin level be detected?

a. 10-12 hours
b. 2-3 hours
c. 5-10 minutes
d. 2-3 days

81. Your patient is found to have an increased calcium level. What is one possible cause of this lab value?

a. Hypoparathyroidism
b. Hyperthyroidism
c. Hypoalbuminemia
d. Hypothyroidism

82. You are educating a patient who has just been diagnosed with cytomegalovirus (CMV). Which of the following statements is correct regarding the patient's condition?

   a. CMV is usually contracted late in life
   b. CMV is easily curable
   c. CMV can often mimic mononucleosis
   d. CMV is often contracted through skin-to-skin contact

83. Your patient's lab results show a low hemoglobin and low hematocrit. Which of the following statements are true regarding these 2 values?

   a. They do not correlate with each other in any way
   b. The hemoglobin value is often 3 times the value of the hematocrit
   c. These labs are usually drawn as part of the basic metabolic panel (BMP)
   d. The hematocrit value is often 3 times the value of the hemoglobin

84. A 58-year-old morbidly obese patient admitted to your unit has a history of hyperlipidemia (high cholesterol). Which of the following lab results is most likely responsible for this condition?

a. Decreased LDL
b. Decreased HDL
c. Decreased VLDL
d. Decreased total cholesterol

85. Which of the following lab values would most likely indicate that the patient is at an increased risk for infection?

a. Low CD4 count
b. High CD4 count
c. Low D-diner
d. High D-dimer

86. You are caring for a patient who has been admitted for a sickle cell crisis. This disorder is characterized by the abnormal appearance of the red blood cells (RBCs), most resembling which of the following shapes?

a. Square
b. Circle
c. Crescent
d. Oval

87. The doctor has ordered an arterial blood gas (ABG) to assess the patient's respiratory status. You know that a normal pH level is in which range?

a. 7.05-7.15
b. 7.35-7.45
c. 6.35-6.45
d. 7.55-7.65

88. Which lab value would most likely be increased in the patient with congestive heart failure (CHF)?

    a. Atrial Natriuretic Peptide (ANP)
    b. Red Blood Cells (RBCs)
    c. Blood Urea Nitrogen (BUN)
    d. Bilirubin

89. A patient with liver disease is shown to have an increased bilirubin. The nurse knows that indirect bilirubin is made up of, in part, from which substance in the body?

    a. White Blood Cells
    b. Hemoglobin
    c. Saliva
    d. Urine

90. Triglycerides are an important component when evaluating cholesterol levels. Before excess triglycerides are deposited into fatty tissue, what is their main function?

    a. Fight infection
    b. Store energy
    c. Increase blood volume
    d. Increase gastric motility

91. Which of the following electrolytes is the main cation on the inside of the cells?

    a. Potassium
    b. Sodium
    c. Magnesium
    d. Chloride

92. A 22 year-old male patient with type 1 diabetes was found down by a family member and is in diabetic ketoacidosis (DKA). Which of the following lab values would the nurse be most concerned with while treating this condition?

    a. Hemoglobin
    b. Triglycerides
    c. Anion Gap
    d. C-reactive protein

93. Which of the following lab results is a common finding in a patient with liver disease?

    a. Decreased Aspartate Aminotransferase (AST, SGOT)
    b. Decreased Prothrombin Time (PT)
    c. Increased Platelet Count (Plts)
    d. Increased Aspartate Aminotransferase (AST, SGOT)

94. Your patient with growth hormone (GH, HGH) deficiency would like to know more about their condition. You know that growth hormone is secreted from which of the following?

    a. Posterior pituitary gland
    b. Adrenal glands
    c. Anterior pituitary gland
    d. Thyroid gland

95. A 79-year-old female with a history of atrial flutter is admitted for possible Coumadin (warfarin) toxicity. Her gums bleed when brushing her teeth, and she now has epistaxis that she has been unable to control. Which of the following medications can be given to counteract the effects of the Coumadin?

a. Vitamin K
b. Potassium
c. Heparin
d. Vitamin D

96. A patient who is post-op day 3 from a laparoscopic ascending colon resection has become hypotensive and tachycardic, with a fever of 102.5 F. The attending physician has ordered a lactic acid level to be drawn. Which of the following conditions is the most likely to be diagnosed if this lab value is elevated?

a. Anemia
b. Congestive heart failure
c. Sepsis
d. Dehydration

97. A patient who is 32 weeks pregnant has been admitted to the labor and delivery unit with severe preeclampsia. When medications fail to bring the blood pressure down to an acceptable level, the physician is concerned that the baby may have to be delivered early. An L/S (lecithin/sphingomyelin) ratio is ordered, a test that primarily checks for which of the following?

a. Brain maturity of the fetus
b. Heart maturity of the fetus
c. Kidney maturity of the fetus
d. Lung maturity of the fetus

98. Your patient with atrial fibrillation is on chronic Coumadin therapy. Which lab value would you expect to be increased because of this medication?

a. Hematocrit
b. Platelets
c. Troponin
d. INR

99. Release of the Parathyroid hormone (PTH) can be stimulated by which of the following?

a. Low sodium
b. Low potassium
c. Low calcium
d. High potassium

100.   Your patient has been placed on an IV heparin drip after being diagnosed with a DVT in the right leg. Which of the following lab values would be most appropriate to monitor the effectiveness of the heparin?

a. Thromboelastography (TEG)
b. Atrial Natriuretic Peptide (ANP)
c. Brain Natriuretic Peptide (BNP)
d. Partial Thromboplastin Time (PTT)

101.   Which of the following lab tests would most likely indicate that liver damage is present?

a. Low Creatinine
b. High Alanine Aminotransferase (ALT, SGPT)
c. Low Alanine Aminotransferase (ALT, SGPT)
d. High Creatinine

102.   A 48-year-old female admitted after a total knee replacement is found to have an increased alkaline phosphatase (ALP, Alk Phos). The nurse knows that this may indicate which of the following conditions? Select all that apply.

a. Hypothyroidism
b. Liver disease
c. Sarcoidosis
d. Pernicious anemia
e. Myocardial infarction
f. Paget disease

103.　　You are monitoring an 84-year-old patient from an assisted living facility, who has just been admitted to the medical-surgical floor. When reviewing the lab results, you note that the albumin level is low. This would most likely indicate which of the following conditions?

a. Dehydration
b. Malnutrition
c. Dementia
d. Fibromyalgia

104.　　While treating a patient in diabetic ketoacidosis (DKA), you are unable to find the anion gap in the lab report. What is one way to calculate the anion gap using other lab values?

a. Chloride – (sodium + bicarbonate)
b. Troponin + (Creatinine – BUN)
c. Hemoglobin - hematocrit
d. Sodium – (chloride + bicarbonate)

105.   The patient has increased amylase and lipase levels. The nurse is aware that the following condition is most likely to result in this finding:

a. Pancreatitis
b. Cardiomyopathy
c. Nephritis
d. Diverticulitis

106.   You are caring for a 47-year-old male with end-stage renal disease, on hemodialysis 3 days a week. When you look at the monitor, you notice that he is in normal sinus rhythm, but the T waves are much higher than normal (peaked). Which of the following lab values is the most likely cause for this reading?

a. Hypokalemia
b. Hyponatremia
c. Hyperkalemia
d. Hypernatremia

107.   Which of the following lab values would you expect to see included in a complete blood count (CBC)?

a. Glucose
b. Hematocrit
c. Alanine aminotransferase (ALT)
d. Lipase

108.   The nurse is assessing a patient with Addison Disease. Which of the following areas of the body is responsible for releasing Adrenocorticotropic Hormone (ACTH)?

a. Posterior pituitary gland
b. Thymus
c. Pineal gland
d. Anterior pituitary gland

109.   Your patient with alcoholic cirrhosis is becoming progressively confused and somnolent. The doctor on call has ordered lactulose to be started immediately. Which lab value would you most likely expect to be increased in this scenario?

a. Creatinine
b. Hematocrit
c. Platelets
d. Ammonia

110.   Red blood cells (RBCs) are a vital component to the function of the body. The nurse knows that they are produced in which of the following?

a. Smooth muscle
b. Bone marrow
c. Small intestine
d. Skeletal muscle

NCLEX-Style Practice Questions with Answers and Rationales

This section shows the 110 NCLEX-style lab value questions with the correct answers and rationales for each. If you'd prefer to test yourself first, go back to the previous section on page 153.

1. The patient has had a cough with blood-tinged sputum for 3 weeks. During differential diagnosis, the nurse knows that which of the following tests may be ordered to help rule out tuberculosis?

   a. Carcinoembryonic Antigen (CEA)
   b. **Acid-Fact Bacillus (AFB)**
   c. Coombs Test
   d. Cytomegalovirus (CMV)

Correct Answer: B

Rationale: An AFB smear will tell you if the patient has the same bacteria that is present in tuberculosis, but it won't give a definitive diagnosis. An AFB culture may take 6-8 weeks, but can usually confirm whether or not the patient has tuberculosis. A CEA is done to screen for cancer and a Coombs test is utilized primarily during cross-matching of blood. CMV is an infection unrelated to tuberculosis.

2. The nurse has been made aware of the patient's increased Activated Clotting Time (ACT). In which of the following scenarios would this be an expected finding? Choose all that apply.

   a. **Heparin therapy**
   b. Thrombosis
   c. **Liver Disease**
   d. **Coumadin therapy**
   e. Psoriasis
   f. Myocardial Infarction

   Correct Answer: A, C, D

   Rationale: When a patient's ACT is increased, they are more prone to bleeding. Heparin, liver disease, and coumadin can all cause the ACT to increase. Thrombosis is a clot, which is very uncommon when the ACT is increased. Psoriasis is a skin condition unrelated to the ACT. A myocardial infarction happens when a blood clot blocks blood flow to the heart. The higher the ACT, the less likely a clot will occur.

3. The nurse knows that the Brain Natriuretic Peptide (BNP) is an important lab result to follow in a patient with congestive heart failure (CHF). Which area of the body is this substance released from?

   a. **Ventricles of the heart**
   b. Atria of the heart
   c. Left lower lobe of the lungs
   d. Right middle lobe of the lungs

   Correct Answer: A

   Rationale: BNP is released from the ventricles of the heart, whereas ANP is released from the atria of the heart.

4. The student nurse is taking care of an 83-year-old male on hemodialysis. Which of the following statements indicates the need for further teaching?

a. It is common for the creatinine to be *increased* in patients with kidney disease
b. Blood Urea Nitrogen (BUN) is commonly *increased* in patients with kidney disease
c. **Blood Urea Nitrogen (BUN) is commonly *decreased* in patients with kidney disease**
d. It is common for the potassium to be *increased* in patients with kidney disease

Correct Answer: C

Rationale: Creatinine, BUN, and potassium are all more likely to be increased in patients with kidney disease. When the kidneys are not working properly, they are unable to filter these substances adequately into the urine.

5. While reviewing lab values, the nurse knows it is more important to pay attention to the ionized calcium, since the total calcium can be affected by which of the following?

a. Bilirubin
b. Ammonia
c. **Albumin**
d. Erythrocytes

Correct Answer: C

Rationale: Total calcium includes protein-bound calcium and ionized calcium. Calcium that is bound to protein is dependent on that protein, which consists mostly of albumin. Because of that, total calcium can be affected by the patient's albumin level. If the albumin is low, then calcium won't have as much protein to bind to, and will therefore be lower.

6. You tap on your patient's facial nerve in an attempt to elicit a contraction response of the facial muscles. When the patient asks what you are doing, the most appropriate response would be which of the following?

   a. I am checking for Chvostek's sign to see if you may have a *high* calcium level
   b. **I am checking for Chvostek's sign to see if you may have a *low* calcium level**
   c. I am checking for Trousseau's sign to see if you may have a *high* calcium level
   d. I am checking for Trousseau's sign to see if you may have a *low* calcium level

Correct Answer: B

Rationale: When a patient has a low calcium level, it may elicit a positive Chvostek's sign or Trousseau's sign. Chvostek's sign is when the facial muscles contract after tapping on the facial nerve. Trousseau's sign is when the muscles in the hand and forearm spasm after the brachial artery is occluded for 3 minutes.

7. A 53-year-old male patient was admitted 24 hours ago with a myocardial infarction. The nurse is aware that which of the following lab results is most likely elevated?

a. Glucose
b. BUN
c. INR
d. **CK-MB**

Correct Answer: D

Rationale: CK-MB is a substance that is released when there has been injury to the heart muscle. The lab value will return to normal within 2-3 days unless the damage continues. Glucose, BUN, and INR may all be elevated, but we have no way of knowing that based on the patient's history that is presented. We know there has been damage to the heart, and that's all we know. Therefore, the best answer is CK-MB.

8. Your patient with stage III kidney disease has been prescribed IV antibiotics. Which of the following lab values would be most helpful in identifying the glomerular filtration rate (GFR) and overall kidney function?

   a. Prothrombin time
   b. Creatinine clearance
   c. BUN
   d. Sodium level

Correct Answer: B

Rationale: Creatinine clearance is important to know for certain antibiotics that are excreted and/or metabolized renally. You need a 24-hour urine test to obtain the creatinine clearance, but the GFR can be estimated using blood tests and patient information. The BUN would help in determining kidney function, but is not very useful by itself in identifying the GFR.

9. The patient's lab results show an increased creatinine level. When the preceptor asks what it means, what would be the most appropriate response by the student nurse?

a. **It is usually indicative of kidney disease**
b. It suggests a problem with myocardial function
c. It is usually indicative of liver disease
d. It often means that there is a problem with the pancreas

Correct Answer: A

Rationale: Creatinine is released by skeletal muscle and eliminated by the kidneys. When there is kidney damage, they can't get rid of it as easily, and the serum creatinine will rise. Knowing the creatinine level alone will not reveal myocardial function, liver disease, or pancreatic problems.

10. The patient you are caring for has an elevated LDL level. In which of the following conditions would this lab result be most expected?

a. Hypertension
b. Hyperlipidemia
c. Diabetes
d. Hypothyroidism

Correct Answer: B

Rationale: Low-Density Lipoproteins (LDL), along with HDL, VLDL, and Triglycerides, help to determine the patients cholesterol level. A patient with an increased LDL would most likely have high cholesterol (hyperlipidemia). Although a patient with hyperlipidemia may also have hypertension and diabetes, an increased LDL level doesn't necessarily mean the patient has these problems.

11. The nurse knows that increased total cholesterol can lead to atherosclerosis, which increases the risk for which of the following?

a. Pleural effusion
b. Congestive Heart Failure
c. Liver cirrhosis
d. **Myocardial infarction**

Correct Answer: D

Rationale: Atherosclerosis is the build-up of plaque in the arteries. The more the plaque builds up, the greater the risk of pieces of the plaque breaking off and traveling through the vascular system. If a piece is large enough, it may clog a major artery that leads to an important organ, such as the heart (myocardial infarction).

12. The attending physician has ordered a ventilation/perfusion (V/Q) scan after your patient suddenly started complaining of chest pain and shortness of breath. This test is often performed to rule out which of the following conditions?

a. Myocardial infarction
b. Hepatitis
c. Appendicitis
d. Pulmonary embolism

Correct Answer: D

Rationale: A V/Q scan is a measure of the ventilation (V) and perfusion (Q) ratio to determine the likelihood of a pulmonary embolism being present. A pulmonary embolism will cause a blockage in the blood flow to the lungs, which causes a disruption in the perfusion.

13. Your patient has been admitted for appendicitis, and currently has a fever and tachycardia. Which of the following lab results would you most likely expect in this scenario?

    a. **Increased white blood cell (WBC) count**
    b. Increased red blood cell (RBC) count
    c. Increased prothrombin time (PT)
    d. Decreased prothrombin time (PT)

Correct Answer: A

Rationale: Appendicitis is inflammation of the appendix, and rupture could lead to a serious infection. If the patient has tachycardia and a fever, an infection must be considered. When an infection is present, the white blood cell (WBC) count will usually be increased as the body attempts to fight it off. Also, the WBC count is increased in most cases of appendicitis on its own, rupture or not. There is no reason to think that any of the other listed lab values would be elevated, based on the information presented.

14. Secretion of Atrial Natriuretic Peptide (ANP) would most likely be stimulated in which of the following conditions?

a. **Congestive Heart Failure**
b. Hyponatremia
c. Dehydration
d. Hypotension

Correct Answer: A

Rationale: ANP is released whenever there is an increased amount of blood volume, such as in congestive heart failure (CHF). It works to decrease water and sodium from the body. The other 3 answer choices are counterintuitive to this objective. A patient with hyponatremia, dehydration, or hypotension would not need water or sodium to be decreased.

15. 10 units of regular insulin has been ordered for your patient with type 2 diabetes. Under normal circumstances, which part of the body is insulin secreted from?

a. Alpha cells of the pancreas
b. Anterior pituitary gland
c. **Beta cells of the pancreas**
d. Posterior pituitary

Correct Answer: C

Rationale: Insulin is secreted from the beta cells in the Islet of Langerhans of the pancreas. Glucagon is released from the alpha cells. The pituitary gland has nothing to do with insulin secretion.

16. A patient who was admitted with Lyme disease is concerned about transmitting the disease to his family. You assure him that it is not a contagious disease and is usually transmitted by which of the following?

   a. Deer
   b. Deer ticks
   c. Horse ticks
   d. Fleas

Correct Answer: B

Rationale: Most cases of Lyme disease are transmitted by deer ticks that carry bacteria called Borrelia burgdorferi. Ticks usually have to be attached to some part of the body for at least 1-2 days before transmission can occur.

17. Your patient's lab results show an increased parathyroid hormone (PTH) level. Which of the following conditions may be the cause for this value? Select all that apply.

a. **Hyperparathyroidism**
b. **Hypocalcemia**
c. **Vitamin D deficiency**
d. **Rickets**
e. Hypomagnesemia
f. Hypercalcemia

Correct Answer: A, B, C, D

Rationale: Common causes for an increased PTH include hyperparathyroidism, certain cancers, Rickets, renal disease, hypocalcemia, and vitamin D deficiency. Common causes for a decreased PTH include hypomagnesemia, Graves disease, sarcoidosis, hypercalcemia, hypoparathyroidism, and excessive vitamin D intake.

18. Sickle cell disease is caused by the presence of which of the following?

   a. Hemoglobin A
   b. Hematocrit A
   c. **Hemoglobin S**
   d. Hemoglobin F

Correct Answer: C

Rationale: Sickle cell is a genetic disorder in which the RBCs become misshapen into a crescent-like form instead of its usual round form. This is caused by the presence of Hemoglobin S, rather than the typical Hemoglobin A.

19. You are caring for a patient with B12 deficiency. Which of the following tests is helpful in determining the cause?

a. Coombs test
b. Chvostek's sign
c. Schilling test
d. Trousseau's sign

Correct Answer: C

Rationale: The Schilling test is to find out if vitamin B12 is being absorbed the way it should. The Coombs test is done primarily during blood cross-matching, while Chvostek's and Trousseau's sign are both done for a patient suspected of hypocalcemia.

20. A patient who is being tested for thyroid disease is waiting to review the lab results with the physician. In regards to thyroxine (T4) and triiodothyronine (T3), which of the following statements are true?

a. T3 is more abundant than T4
b. T3 is weaker than T4
c. **T4 is more abundant than T3**
d. T3 and T4 are equal in abundance

Correct Answer: C

Rationale: T4 is weaker than T3, but it is much more abundant. All of the other answer choices are false.

21. While drawing an ABG, the nurse knows that which lab value will most likely cause acidosis?

a. Low PaCO2 *Resp. Alkalosis*
b. High HCO3 *Metabolic Alkalosis*
c. High PaO2 *Resp. Acidosis*
d. **High PaCO2** *Resp. Acidosis*

Correct Answer: D

Rationale: A high PaCO2 and a low HCO3 would most likely cause acidosis. Although the pH may be compensated, it is impossible to know based on the information provided. Therefore, the best answer is high PaCO2. PaO2 is typically irrelevant when it comes to determining pH.

22. Your patient has just arrived back to the unit from the operating room. Initial lab results show a low hemoglobin and hematocrit. The patient is awake, sitting up in bed. Which of the following is the most likely to be ordered to specifically treat this?

a. **Blood products**
b. Broad-spectrum antibiotics
c. Immediate Intubation
d. Fluid restriction

Correct Answer: A

Rationale: A low hemoglobin and hematocrit indicate that the patient may need blood products. Although antibiotics may be needed because of surgery, they won't help a low hemoglobin and hematocrit. The patient is awake and alert, so intubation is not necessary at this time. Fluid restriction would not be wise if these lab values are low. In fact, fluid may need to be given until the blood can be transfused.

23. A 22-year-old female patient is in the emergency room for intractable nausea and vomiting. The attending physician has ordered an hCG level (human chorionic gonadotropin). The nurse knows that which of the following diagnoses are being ruled out?

a. Infection
b. Myocardial Infarction
c. **Pregnancy**
d. Pulmonary Embolism

Correct Answer: C

Rationale: The patient is of child-bearing age and has symptoms common during pregnancy. Pregnancy must be ruled out, which is done by determining the hCG level. The hCG will not reveal any information in regards to the other 3 answer choices.

24. A 33-year-old female who had surgery on her left ankle 2 days ago now has an increased anion gap. This particular lab value is most likely to indicate which of the following conditions?

a. Alkalosis
b. **Acidosis**
c. Increased bicarbonate
d. Decreased hydrogen ions

Correct Answer: B

Rationale: An increased anion gap is indicative of acidosis. This is a common lab finding when a patient is in sepsis, which should be considered after possible infection from surgery. The anion gap is not increased because of alkalosis. Because of this, the other choices would not cause an increase since they would likely lead to alkalosis.

25. Your patient's lab results show a decreased albumin level. After being produced in the liver, what is the main function of albumin?

a. **Maintain the colloidal osmotic pressure**
b. Control blood pressure
c. Maintain sodium balance
d. Control the blood-brain barrier

Correct Answer: A

Rationale: Albumin is the largest component of total protein in the blood. It is produced in the liver and its job is to maintain the colloidal osmotic pressure. This pressure makes sure that fluid is balanced between the tissues in the body and the capillaries. When there is a problem, water can leak out into the tissue, causing edema.

26. Your patient's lab results reveal an elevated bilirubin level. In which condition is this most likely related to?

a. Renal failure
b. Hepatitis
c. Pulmonary edema
d. Colitis

Correct Answer: B

Rationale: Bilirubin makes up a major portion of bile. When the liver has a hard time getting rid of the bilirubin, it begins to build up in the body and can cause jaundice (a yellowish discoloration of the skin). If the reason for the build-up is due to a liver disorder, then the indirect bilirubin will be increased. If the issue lies beyond the liver, as is the case with gallstones and blocked bile ducts, then the direct bilirubin will be increased. However, it has nothing to do with renal failure, pulmonary edema, or colitis. Therefore, the best answer is hepatitis, which is a disorder of the liver.

27. As a nurse, it is important to know which labs will be included with each panel that is ordered. Which of the following lab panels would include the alanine aminotransferase (ALT, SGPT) level?

a. Complete blood count (CBC)
b. Basic metabolic panel (BMP)
c. Renal Panel
d. **Comprehensive metabolic panel (CMP)**

Correct Answer: D

Rationale: A CBC includes the white blood count, hemoglobin, hematocrit, and platelets. A BMP includes sodium, potassium, chloride, CO2, BUN, creatinine, and glucose. A renal panel includes the BUN, creatinine, electrolytes, proteins, and minerals. A CMP is the correct answer because it includes everything the BMP has, plus proteins, calcium, and liver function tests, including the ALT.

28. Your patient has been diagnosed with Syndrome of Inappropriate ADH Secretion (SIADH). In which part of the body does production of ADH occur?

a. Adrenal glands
b. Thyroid gland
c. **Hypothalamus**
d. Parathyroid gland

Correct Answer: C

Rationale: ADH is stored in the posterior pituitary gland, but is produced in the hypothalamus. The other 3 answer choices are unrelated.

29. A patient you are caring for is in Hyperglycemic Hyperosmolar Nonketotic Coma (HHNK). Which of the following lab values would you most likely expect to see?

a. Low glucose
b. High creatinine
c. Low creatinine
d. **High glucose**

Correct Answer: D

Rationale: HHNK is a condition that is seen when glucose gets too high in diabetics, usually type II. Therefore, the most likely lab to be elevated is the glucose.

30. Which of the following scenarios is the most likely cause of an increased C-reactive protein (CRP)?

a. **An infected wound**
b. Parkinson's disease
c. Alzheimer's disease
d. A steroid injection

Correct Answer: A

Rationale: An increased C-reactive protein is indicative of inflammation and/or infection somewhere in the body. Parkinson's and Alzheimer's are unrelated, and a steroid injection may actually cause a decrease in this lab value.

31. Your patient's erythrocyte sedimentation rate (ESR) is elevated. Which of the following is incorrect regarding this lab result?

a. **It is a very specific diagnostic tool**
b. It may be elevated during infection
c. It is often elevated during inflammation
d. It measures the rate at which RBCs settle in a solution over time

Correct Answer: A

Rationale: The ESR is a very non-specific tool. It is elevated when there is inflammation and/or infection somewhere in the body, but cannot pinpoint an exact location.

32. A 53-year-old female has arrived at the doctor's office to review her most recent lab results. Every result is close to the normal range, with the exception of the follicle-stimulating hormone (FSH), which is elevated. Which of the following conditions may cause an elevated FSH? Select all that apply.

a. Malnutrition
b. **Pituitary tumor**
c. **Menopause**
d. **Polycystic ovaries**
e. Pregnancy

Correct Answer: B, C, D

Rationale: Possible causes for an increased FSH include menopause, pituitary tumor, castration, polycystic ovaries, puberty, and testicular damage. Possible causes for a decreased FSH include malnutrition, stress, pituitary failure, and pregnancy.

33. You notice that your patient's lab results include an increased sodium level. Which of the following symptoms would they most likely present in relation to hypernatremia?

a. Excessive hunger
b. Clear urine
c. Fever
d. **Excessive thirst**

Correct Answer: D

Rationale: Cardinal signs of hypernatremia include edema and excessive thirst. Typically, urine is clear if hydration is adequate, which is unlikely in cases of hypernatremia. The other 2 choices are unrelated.

34. You are caring for a 47-year old male with lung cancer, who has been receiving chemotherapy for the last 6 months. The most recent lab results show a decreased white blood cell count. This puts the patient at an increased risk for which of the following?

a. **Infection**
b. Blood loss
c. Muscle loss
d. Muscle cramps

Correct Answer: A

Rationale: Patients who are on chemotherapy often have a low WBC count, putting them at a higher risk for infection. These patients are typically placed on neutropenic precautions, in which steps are taken to avoid transmission of illnesses from staff and visitors.

35. In a patient who is suspected to have tuberculosis, which of the following statements is correct?

a. An AFB smear is more sensitive than an AFB culture

b. **An AFB smear will yield results much faster than an AFB culture** Acid- Fast Bacillus

c. An AFB smear is a definitive diagnosis of tuberculosis

d. The most common body fluid to be tested for an AFB smear is urine

Correct Answer: B

Rationale: An AFB smear will typically yield results within a few hours, whereas an AFB culture could take 6-8 weeks. However, a culture is much more sensitive. Sputum is the typical body fluid to be tested.

36. You are caring for a patient who has been admitted for surgery related to a positive BRCA test. Which of the following surgeries would you most likely expect to be done?

a. Craniotomy
b. Mastectomy
c. Splenectomy
d. Vasectomy

Correct Answer: B

Rationale: A positive BRCA test indicates that the patient has an increased risk for developing breast cancer. When this happens, it is recommended that prophylactic mastectomies be performed.

37. You are caring for a patient who is being treated for deep vein thrombosis (DVT). Which of the following disorders would cause the greatest risk for blood clots?

    a. Heterozygous Factor V Leiden
    b. Thrombocytopenia
    c. **Homozygous Factor V Leiden**
    d. Liver cirrhosis

Correct Answer: C

Rationale: Factor V Leiden increases the risk for developing blood clots. Patients with the homozygous form of the disease are much more at risk than those with the heterozygous form. Thrombocytopenia and liver cirrhosis will typically decrease the risk for blood clots.

38. The patient was found unresponsive at home by a family member. The family member states that the power was off and a generator was running in the living room when he got there. The patient stopped breathing by the time the paramedics arrived, but the oxygen saturation was 100%. Which lab value would you expect to be increased when the patient gets to the hospital?

a. **Carbon Monoxide (CO)**
b. PaO2
c. Hemoglobin
d. Hematocrit

Correct Answer: A

Rationale: This is a classic case of carbon monoxide poisoning, commonly happening after running a generator indoors. The oxygen saturation may still read 100% even if the patient is hypoxic. This is because pulse oximetry measures oxygenated blood, not differentiating between oxygen (O2) and carbon monoxide (CO).

39. Your patient's lab results revealed an increased carcinoembryonic antigen (CEA) level. This is indicative of which of the following?

a. It always means cancer is present
b. It never means cancer is present
c. **It may be caused by more than just cancer**
d. It can only be caused by cancer

Correct Answer: C

Rationale: Although an increased CEA often indicates that cancer is present, that isn't always the case. It may also be increased in Chron's disease, cirrhosis, peptic ulcers, and inflammatory conditions.

40. A morbidly obese patient is admitted to your unit. The lab results show an elevated D-Dimer level. This typically indicates that the patient has a greater chance of which of the following risks?

a. Liver damage
b. infection
c. Diabetes
d. **Blood clots**

Correct Answer: D

Rationale: The D-dimer measures plasmin and thrombin activity. When these are high, there is a greater chance of the blood clotting. It is also tested to check for the effectiveness of anticoagulant therapy. If there was liver damage, chances are the patient would be more prone to bleeding, not clotting. The other 2 answer choices are irrelevant.

41. Lactate Dehydrogenase (LDH) may be drawn to detect which of the following conditions?

a. High cholesterol
b. Specific tissue damage or infection
c. **Generalized tissue damage or infection**
d. Certain sexually-transmitted diseases

Correct Answer: C

Rationale: LDH is a substance that is in the cells of most of the tissues in the body. When these cells are damaged, the LDH is released into the bloodstream, causing an increase in the lab value. The problem is that it is very hard to pinpoint where the damage is because it can be found in so many places. LDH may rise in certain types of anemia, infection, kidney or liver disease, broken bones, some cancers, and muscle injuries. Sometimes this lab is drawn in cerebrospinal fluid (CSF) to differentiate between bacterial and viral meningitis (high LDH usually points to bacterial). It may also be tested from pleural, peritoneal, and pericardial fluid to help diagnose certain problems, such as liver cirrhosis and CHF.

42. Which of the following tests would be the most sensitive when trying to confirm the diagnosis of tuberculosis?

a. Blood culture
b. **AFB Culture** — Acid- Fast Bacillus
c. AFB smear
d. Rapid strep test

Correct Answer: B

Rationale: An AFB smear will typically yield results within a few hours, whereas an AFB culture could take 6-8 weeks. However, a culture is much more sensitive.

43. A 62-year-old male has arrived to the ER by ambulance, complaining of chest pain. The care team is concerned that the patient is having a myocardial infarction, and begin appropriate treatment measures. Which of the following lab values would most likely be elevated in this scenario?

a. INR
b. Glucose
c. **Troponin**
d. Creatinine

Correct Answer: C

Rationale: Troponin is increased whenever there is injury to the myocardium, which would be the case in a myocardial infarction. It is impossible to know if the other lab values are elevated based on the information.

44. In which of the following conditions would you expect your patient's adrenocorticotropic hormone (ACTH) to be elevated?

a. Long-term steroid use
b. Secondary Adrenal insufficiency
c. **Addison disease**
d. Hypopituitarism

Correct Answer: C

Rationale: ACTH is increased in Addison Disease, Cushing Syndrome/Disease, and stress. ACTH is decreased in patients with an adrenal adenoma, chronic steroid use, secondary adrenal insufficiency, and hypopituitarism.

45. Growth hormone (GH) may be decreased in which of the following conditions? Select all that apply?

a. Acromegaly
b. During exercise
c. **Dwarfism**
d. **Pituitary insufficiency**
e. During stress
f. During surgery

Correct Answer: C, D

Rationale: GH is often increased with exercise, Acromegaly, diabetes, anorexia, stress, hypoglycemia, and surgery. GH may be decreased in patients with Dwarfism, GH deficiency, hyperglycemia, pituitary insufficiency, and failure to thrive.

46. Your 43-year-old male patient has been admitted with acute pancreatitis. Which of the following lab values would you expect to be increased because of this condition?

a. **Lipase**
b. Calcium
c. Triglycerides
d. Thyroxine

Correct Answer: A

Rationale: Amylase and lipase are often used to help diagnose pancreatic problems. A patient with pancreatitis would likely have both of these lab values elevated. Calcium, triglycerides, and thyroxine are unrelated.

47. During a code, you notice the patient's rhythm appear to resemble ventricular tachycardia, but with a twisting quality. You suspect that it is torsades de pointes, knowing that this condition is likely caused by which lab value?

a. High magnesium
b. High calcium
c. **Low magnesium**
d. Low calcium

Correct Answer: C

Rationale: Low magnesium is a common cause of a lethal arrhythmia called torsades de pointes, which means "twisting of the points." It is a type of ventricular tachycardia that appears to be twisting at the QRS complex. This is why you'll see magnesium as a standard part of code carts.

Causes of low magnesium -
Low magnesium is due to ↓ absorption of magnesium in the gut or ↑ excretion of magnesium in the urine. Magnesium levels are largely controlled by the kidneys.
- Diabetes, Poor Absorption, chronic diarrhea, Celiac disease

48. Thromboelastography (TEG) is a fairly new test that would most likely be used to determine which of the following?

[handwritten: measures the quality of platelets, how efficient they're working]

a. **Platelet quality**
b. Hemoglobin quality
c. Hemoglobin count
d. Platelet count

Correct Answer: A

Rationale: Not all platelets are created equally, as some work better than others. Two patients may have identical labs with a platelet count of 100,000, but one will be at a higher risk of bleeding. This is where the TEG comes in. A platelet count will tell you how many platelets there are, but a TEG will show you how efficient those platelets are working.

49. A patient with a decreased Thyroid-stimulating hormone (TSH) level is most likely to have which of the following conditions?

a. Hypothyroidism
b. **Graves disease**
c. Hashimoto's thyroiditis
d. Addison's disease

Correct Answer: B

Rationale: The TSH is used in conjunction with other lab values to help evaluate thyroid function and diagnose thyroid disorders. When a patient has hypothyroidism (decreased function), there is a decrease in T3 and T4. This causes the TSH to rise in an attempt to bring these levels up. Therefore, a high TSH would indicate the possibility of primary hypothyroidism. In patients with Graves disease and other forms of hyperthyroidism, you would find the TSH levels to be low, while at the same time, the T3 and T4 levels would be high.

50. The parathyroid hormone (PTH) is responsible for causing the release of which of the following electrolytes when stimulated?

a. Potassium
b. Sodium
c. Magnesium
d. **Calcium**

Correct Answer: D

Rationale: When the calcium level in the body is low, the parathyroid gland responds by releasing PTH into the bloodstream. It stimulates the osteoclasts in the bone to release calcium and causes the kidneys to reabsorb it, as well as increase the absorption by the GI system.

51. Your patient's body has difficulty absorbing B12. Which of the following disorders would this most likely be associated with?

    a. Iron-deficient anemia
    b. Pernicious anemia
    c. Thrombocytopenia
    d. Leukemia

Correct Answer: B

Rationale: Absorption of B12 usually happens in the ileum of the intestine after combining with intrinsic factor. If any of the B12 isn't needed, it gets sent out of the body in the urine. If there is a problem absorbing the B12, something called pernicious anemia can develop. This happens because B12 is needed to make red blood cells (RBCs). If there's not enough, anemia will occur.

52. Which of the following lab values is the most likely to be increased when there is new bone growth, such as after fracture or during adolescents?

a. Amylase
b. Aspartate aminotransferase (AST)
c. **Alkaline phosphatase (ALP)**
d. D-dimer

Correct Answer: C

Rationale: ALP is a substance found in many places throughout the body, but it's mostly contained in the bone, liver, and biliary tract. This lab is drawn when you want to diagnose disorders in these areas. ALP is also increased more when there is new bone growth. Because of this, you will see a higher level in kids and teenagers. There is also new abnormal bone growth when there is metastasis to the bone, fractures that are healing, rheumatoid arthritis, Paget disease, and hyperparathyroidism.

53. The patient in metabolic alkalosis would most likely have which results on the arterial blood gas (ABG)?

a. pH 7.61, PaCO2 25, HCO3 23
b. pH 7.40, PaCO2 40, HCO3 24
c. **pH 7.58, PaCO2 37, HCO3 32**
d. pH 7.29, PaCO2 37, HCO3 14

Correct Answer: C

Rationale: Alkalosis is characterized as a pH greater than 7.45. We know that it is metabolic in nature because the HCO3 is elevated and the PaCO2 is normal. If it were respiratory alkalosis, the PaCO2 would be lower.

ABG's

① pH - 7.35- 7.45

② PaCO2- 35-45

③ HCO3 - 22-26

④ Pa O2 - 80-100

54. A newborn who was born 24 hours ago has developed a yellowish tint to their skin, known as jaundice. The nurse knows that the increase of which of the following lab values is the most likely cause?

    a. Albumin
    b. Bilirubin
    c. Bicarbonate
    d. Ferritin

Correct Answer: B

Rationale: Bilirubin makes up a major portion of bile. When the liver has a hard time getting rid of the bilirubin, it begins to build up in the body and can cause jaundice (a yellowish discoloration of the skin). In newborns, the liver is often too immature to convert the indirect bilirubin to direct bilirubin. Because of this, the indirect bilirubin will build up, causing jaundice. This is why you will often see newborn babies with a yellow tint to their skin. This is usually not a problem and will resolve itself within a few days. However, it needs to be monitored and treated if necessary. If the bilirubin level gets too high, it can get to the brain, leading to encephalopathy. If this happens, the infant may be difficult to arouse and can even go into a coma.

55. A rapid strep-test is often used in healthcare settings to quickly rule out strep throat. Patients who test positive and are left untreated are at a higher risk for developing which of the following conditions?

a. **Rheumatic fever**
b. Alzheimer's disease
c. Thyroid cancer
d. Diabetes mellitus

Correct Answer: A

Rationale: If strep throat is not treated properly, it may lead to rheumatic fever. This is a very dangerous condition that can cause several problems, including severe damage to the heart. The other answer choices are unrelated to strep throat.

56. Upon reviewing your patient's lab results, you notice that the sodium level is elevated. This is most likely present in which of the following conditions?

    a. Excessive water intake
    b. Low osmolality
    c. Pleural effusion
    d. Dehydration

Correct Answer: D

Rationale: Excessive water intake and low osmolality typically are associated with hyponatremia. Pleural effusion usually means that the body is holding more water than it needs, another sign of hyponatremia. However, when you are dehydrated, the sodium builds up and hypernatremia develops. It is because there is too much solute (sodium) in relation to solvent (water).

57. Which of the following lab values would most likely be expected in a patient who is in disseminated Intravascular Coagulation (DIC)? not able to clot

a. Decreased PT
b. Increased glucose
c. **Increased D-dimer**
d. Increased platelet count

Correct Answer: C

Rationale: A common lab test to help diagnose a patient in DIC is the D-Dimer. In this condition, the clotting factors are in overdrive until they are all used up. An increased PT and a decreased platelet count might also be expected.

58. Antidiuretic hormone (ADH, vasopressin) is a lab value that can be used most effectively to identify which of the following conditions?

a. Diabetes type 1
b. **Diabetes Insipidus** — *very rare - < 20,000 cases per year.*
c. Diabetes type 2
d. Diabetic ketoacidosis (DKA)

Correct Answer: B

Rationale: ADH is constantly secreted to maintain a balance, adjusting with more or less as needed. Sometimes, there isn't enough ADH secretion to maintain this balance. Sometimes, the kidneys ignore the message ADH is sending. When either of these things happen, you get Diabetes Insipidus (DI). If the cause for this is lack of ADH secretion, it is likely a problem with the central neurologic system (tumor, trauma, etc). This would be known as neurogenic DI. If the problem is with the kidneys, it is known as nephrogenic DI. In either case, you will see large amounts of diluted urine (Low osmolality) and highly concentrated fluid in the body (High osmolality).

Diabetes Insipidus -
A disorder of salt & water metabolism marked by intense thirst & heavy urination.
D.I. Occurs when the body can't regulate how it handles fluids. The condition is a hormonal abnormality & isn't related to diabetes.

265

59. You are taking care of a 65-year-old female with COPD who has smoked a pack of cigarettes per day for 45 years. The arterial blood gas (ABG) shows a pH of 7.29, PaCO2 of 58, and HCO3 of 24. What is the most appropriate classification for these results?

pH ↓

PaCO2 ↑

HCO3 24-nl

a. **Respiratory Acidosis**
b. Respiratory Alkalosis
c. Normal ABG
d. Metabolic Acidosis

Correct Answer: A

Rationale: The pH is below 7.35, so right away we know it is acidosis. The PaCO2 is high, indicating that the problem lies in the respiratory system. The HCO3 is in a normal range, so it isn't able to compensate. If the HCO3 were low, you might consider metabolic as the cause for acidosis.

60. Your patient has a chronically low phosphate (PO4) level. Which of the following conditions is the most likely contributing factor to this?

a. **Chronic antacid intake**
b. Hypocalcemia
c. Hypoparathyroidism
d. Acromegaly

Correct Answer: A

Rationale: High phosphate levels are seen in renal disease, anemia, lymphoma, acidosis, Acromegaly, hypoparathyroidism, hypocalcemia, sarcoidosis, and liver disease. You may see a decreased phosphate level with chronic antacid intake, hyperparathyroidism, sepsis, alkalosis, rickets, malnutrition, hypercalcemia, vitamin D deficiency, and DKA.

61. A 29-year-old female with non-Hodgkin's lymphoma is admitted for a port placement. She has been getting chemotherapy treatments for the past 2 weeks. Her most recent lab results show a very low platelet count, putting her most at risk for which of the following?

a. Blood clots
b. **Excessive Bleeding**
c. Myocardial infarction
d. Cerebrovascular accident

Correct Answer: B

Rationale: As the platelet count gets lower, the harder it is for the body to clot, putting the patient at risk for bleeding. All of the other answer choices point to problems related to clotting.

62. A patient who was admitted 3 hours ago on the medical-surgical floor is found to have an increased Blood Urea Nitrogen (BUN). What are the most common causes of this lab result? Select all that apply.

a. **Kidney Disease**
b. Hypervolemia
c. **Dehydration**
d. COPD
e. **Urinary tract obstruction**
f. **Hemorrhagic shock**

Correct Answer: A, C, E, F

Rationale: BUN may be elevated in kidney disease, dehydration, sepsis, burns, GI bleeds, CHF, urinary tract obstructions, shock, and with certain medications.

63. A 28-year-old female who is being seen in the office is concerned about her family history of cancer. Which of the following lab tests might be helpful in determining her likelihood of developing breast cancer?

a. CNCR
b. BRCA
c. ACTH
d. RISK

Correct Answer: B

Rationale: BRCA is a test to determine risk for developing breast cancer. It is often done in patients with a family history of breast cancer. If the test shows positive, prophylactic mastectomy is recommended.

64. Your patient has a history of congestive heart failure (CHF), and has been admitted with shortness of breath. Which lab value would you most likely expect to find?

a. Increased Alaline Transaminase (ALT, SGPT)
b. Decreased Aspartate Transaminase (AST, SGOT)
c. Decreased Brain Natriuretic Peptide (BNP)
d. **Increased Brain Natriuretic Peptide (BNP)**

Correct Answer: D

Rationale: ALT and AST are labs used to determine liver function. BNP is released whenever the heart is stretched beyond a certain point, such as in fluid overload. This is a common lab used to help diagnose and monitor CHF.

65. Your patient was diagnosed with Human Immunodeficiency Virus (HIV) 5 years ago. Which of the following lab results will indicate how much the disease has progressed since that time?

a. **CD4 Count**
b. Amylase
c. BRCA
d. Fibrinogen

Correct Answer: A

Rationale: As HIV progresses, the CD4 count gets lower and lower without treatment. This will eventually lead to AIDS when the count gets very low (below 200). As the CD4 count drops, it increases the risk for infection. Infections and complications from AIDS are what eventually lead to death. CD4 counts, in combination with other labs, help in keeping track of HIV's progression and guide treatment.

66. You are caring for a patient who just had major abdominal surgery. The doctor has ordered for 2 units of packed red blood cells (PRBCs) to be given. What is one way the blood bank can determine if antibodies are present in the patient's blood sample before transfusing any products?

a. Arterial blood gas (ABG)
b. Blood culture
c. **Coombs test**
d. Hemoglobin A1C

Correct Answer: C

Rationale: During cross-matching, it is important to determine not only the blood type, but also for antibodies which may cause a reaction. This is where the indirect Coombs test comes in. It enables the lab to find out if antibodies are present before the blood is given to a patient.

67. Chloride is an electrolyte that is classified as an anion. The nurse knows that this means it has which of the following properties?

a. Positive charge
b. **Negative charge**
c. Neutral charge
d. No charge

Correct Answer: B

Rationale: An anion has a negative charge, while a cation has a positive. This is easy to remember, because the 't' in the word 'cation' looks like a plus sign (positive).

68. A 29-year-old female, who is 39 weeks pregnant, has been admitted to the labor and delivery unit. When going through her history, she states that she was once told she has an increased risk for blood clots. Which of the following lab values would correlate with this description?

a. Increased PTT
b. **Presence of Factor V Leiden**
c. Thrombocytopenia
d. Iron-deficiency anemia

Correct Answer: B

Rationale: Factor V Leiden is a genetic disorder that increases the risk of developing blood clots. An increased PTT, thrombocytopenia, and anemia would all put the patient at an increased risk of bleeding.

69. Under normal circumstances, red blood cells (RBCs) have a lifespan of how long?

a. **4 months**
b. 4 weeks
c. 4 years
d. 4 hours

Correct Answer: A

Rationale: The RBC is drawn as a part of the CBC (Complete Blood Count). It measures the amount of red blood cells per 1 mm³ that are in venous blood. They are produced in the bone marrow and contain hemoglobin molecules that transport oxygen and carbon dioxide throughout the body. When there are no problems present, a red blood cell can typically survive for 120 days (4 months).

70. A patient with suspected carbon monoxide poisoning has just arrived via ambulance to the emergency room. She is stable and breathing, but very tired and confused. Which of the following treatment options would be the most helpful in this situation?

a. **Oxygen via non-rebreathing mask**
b. IV epinephrine
c. Raising the head of the bed
d. Pain medication

Correct Answer: A

Rationale: The first and most important treatment for carbon monoxide poisoning is oxygen. Although raising the head may help, oxygen should happen first. Pain medication probably wouldn't be a good idea since the patient is already tired and confused. There is no reason to use epinephrine on a stable patient.

71. A 23-year-old female is 7 months pregnant and has been having some abdominal pain and cramping. The obstetrician would like to determine the fetus' Lecithin/Sphingomyelin ratio. Which body fluid would you expect to be tested?

a. Fetal blood
b. Mother's blood
c. Mother's Urine
d. **Amniotic fluid**

Correct Answer: D

Rationale: The L/S Ratio is used to test how well the lungs of a fetus have matured. The sample is taken from the amniotic fluid, a process called an amniocentesis. Surfactant is a very important substance that allows the lungs to work properly, but is even more vital for premature babies. Lecithin (L) and Sphingomyelin (S) are a big part of the make-up of surfactant. The L/S ratio helps to determine the risks and benefits of delivering a baby prematurely. The higher the ratio, the better.

72. Which of the following lab values would you most likely expect to see on an arterial blood gas (ABG) in a patient who is in diabetic ketoacidosis (DKA)?

a. Increased pH
b. Decreased PaCO2
c. Increased base excess (BE)
d. **Decreased HCO3**

Correct Answer: D

Rationale: A patient in DKA would be acidotic, and metabolic in nature. Therefore, you would expect to see a decreased pH and a decreased HCO3. Base excess would likely be decreased also. PaCO2 may be somewhat decreased if the respiratory system is trying to compensate, but this is not always the case.

73. Your patient with type I diabetes begins to feel weak and tired, and appears pale and diaphoretic. Alteration in which of the following labs is the most likely cause of these symptoms?

a. Hemoglobin
b. White blood cells
c. Potassium
d. **Glucose**

Correct Answer: D

Rationale: These symptoms in a diabetic patient strongly suggest hypoglycemia. The other answer choices may indeed be altered, but it's not as likely that they would cause these symptoms in a patient with this history.

74. A patient is being educated on Glucose-6-phosphate-dehydrogenase (G6PD) deficiency. Which of the following statements would indicate that further teaching is required?

a. **It is a genetic y-linked disorder**
b. It is a condition in which the red blood cells may become damaged
c. It is commonly triggered by infection, stress, and certain drugs and foods
d. Men are more likely to inherit the disorder

Correct Answer: A

Rationale: G6PD is an enzyme that aids in the function of red blood cells. When a patient doesn't have enough of this enzyme, the red blood cells may start to get destroyed (hemolysis). It is an X-linked trait, meaning that men are more likely to have it. Women who have the deficiency often have no symptoms.

75. You have decided to test for Trousseau's sign in a patient with hypocalcemia. Which of the following methods would best demonstrate this?

a. Occlude the radial artery for 3 minutes
b. Tap on the patient's cheek
c. **Occlude the brachial artery for 3 minutes**
d. Tap on the patient's palm

Correct Answer: C

Rationale: Patients with hypocalcemia may develop muscle spasms (tetany). You can check for this by assessing your patient for Chvostek's or Trousseau's sign. Chvostek's sign is when the facial muscles contract after tapping on the facial nerve. Trousseau's sign is when the muscles in the hand and forearm spasm after the brachial artery is occluded for 3 minutes (Usually accomplished by inflating a blood pressure cuff higher than the systolic pressure.

The brachial artery is the major blood vessel of the upper arm. It is the continuation of the axillary artery

ulna - pinky side
Radius - thumb (rotates)

282

76. In an environment of anaerobic metabolism, which lab value is the most likely to be increased?

a. PaO2
b. Phosphorus (PO4)
c. **Lactic acid**
d. Hemoglobin

Correct Answer: C

Rationale: The 2 main types of metabolism are aerobic and anaerobic. The body likes to function on aerobic metabolism, in which there is plenty of oxygen available for the tissues. In this state, glucose gets metabolized to CO2 and H2O. Anaerobic metabolism happens when the amount of oxygen to the tissues decreases. Glucose then gets metabolized to lactic acid, rather than CO2. As the lactate increases more and more, patients can develop lactic acidosis.

77. Your diabetic patient has had a consistently high glucose since admission 2 days ago. He states that his blood sugar is usually under control. Which of the following lab tests would be the most helpful in determining how well his diabetes has been controlled over the past 6 months?

a. Glucose-6-Phosphate-Dehydrogenase (G6PD)
b. **Glycated Hemoglobin (HbA1c)**
c. Factor V Leiden
d. Arterial blood gas (ABG)

Correct Answer: B

Rationale: Glycated Hemoglobin is a test most commonly used to see how well patients have controlled their diabetes over a long-term period of time (about 3-4 months). HbA1c is a component of hemoglobin that combines with glucose stronger than any other component. An RBC has a life-span of around 4 months, which is why this test is able to tell what the glucose levels have been in that timeframe. If the level is greater than 6-7%, it can indicate that treatment is not effective or that the patient has not been keeping their sugars under control.

78. You are caring for a patient with severe malnutrition and failure to thrive. The lab results show a decreased total protein, which is comprised of which 2 substances?

a. **Albumin and globulin**
b. Albumin and sodium
c. Bile and globulin
d. Albumin and bile

Correct Answer: A

Rationale: Total protein is an indicator of the overall nutritional status of a patient. Albumin, along with globulin, makes up most of the total protein in the body.

79. A patient who is on chronic Coumadin (warfarin) therapy is likely to have an increase in INR. The INR is derived from which of the following lab values, which is also likely to be elevated?

a. Hemoglobin
b. Platelets
c. Hematocrit
d. **Prothrombin time**

Correct Answer: D

Rationale: The PT is a lab value that is used to assess how well the body is clotting, and therefore the risk of bleeding. The INR is derived from the PT, so these lab values are usually evaluated together. It gauges the effectiveness of the extrinsic and the common pathways of the coagulation cascade. The longer the PT is, the greater the risk of bleeding is (or the greater the anticoagulant therapy is working).

Normal INR Levels - 2.0-3.0

higher INR = ↑ bleeding - blood coagulates too slow

lower INR = ↑ clots / stroke - not thin enough

80. When a patient has a myocardial infarction, how soon can the increased troponin level be detected?

a. 10-12 hours
b. **2-3 hours**
c. 5-10 minutes
d. 2-3 days

Correct Answer: B

Rationale: When a patient has a heart attack, troponin is released into the bloodstream and can be detected within 2-3 hours, and will continue to rise as long as injury is still occurring. Once a troponin is found to be elevated, doctors will usually order serial labs drawn to check the extent of injury and know when it has stopped. When the troponin gets to its highest level, it is said to have "peaked" before it begins its decent back down to normal. It can stay high for up to 2 weeks after an attack.

81. Your patient is found to have an increased calcium level. What is one possible cause of this lab value?

a. Hypoparathyroidism
b. Hyperthyroidism
c. Hypoalbuminemia
d. Hypothyroidism

Correct Answer: B

Rationale: Increased calcium levels may be seen in patients with hyperthyroidism, hyperparathyroidism, Addison Disease, lymphoma, Paget Disease, sarcoidosis, TB, and with certain cancers. You may see a drop in calcium in hypoparathyroidism, hypoalbuminemia, alkalosis, renal failure, pancreatitis, fat embolism, vitamin D deficiency, rickets, and malabsorption.

82. You are educating a patient who has just been diagnosed with cytomegalovirus (CMV). Which of the following statements is correct regarding the patient's condition?

a. CMV is usually contracted late in life
b. CMV is easily curable
c. **CMV can often mimic mononucleosis**
d. CMV is often contracted through skin-to-skin contact

Correct Answer: C

Rationale: CMV is a type of virus that is most often contracted before birth or as a young child, but can occur at any time. You can contract such infections through body fluids and blood transfusions. Unfortunately, there is no cure and can come and go as it pleases. Usually, it stays inactive unless your immune system is compromised. It is not uncommon for there to be no symptoms. If there are symptoms, it can often mimic mononucleosis. You might see fever, stomach ulcers, diarrhea, seizures, blindness, pneumonia, or hepatitis. In very extreme cases, encephalitis and even coma may happen.

83. Your patient's lab results show a low hemoglobin and low hematocrit. Which of the following statements are true regarding these 2 values?

   a. They do not correlate with each other in any way
   b. The hemoglobin value is often 3 times the value of the hematocrit
   c. These labs are usually drawn as part of the basic metabolic panel (BMP)
   d. **The hematocrit value is often 3 times the value of the hemoglobin**

Correct Answer: D

Rationale: These labs are drawn as a part of the complete blood count (CBC), not the basic metabolic panel (BMP). The hematocrit value is often 3 times the value of the hemoglobin. If one goes up, so does the other, and vice versa.

84. A 58-year-old morbidly obese patient admitted to your unit has a history of hyperlipidemia (high cholesterol). Which of the following lab results is most likely responsible for this condition?

a. Decreased LDL
b. Decreased HDL
c. Decreased VLDL
d. Decreased total cholesterol

Correct Answer: B

Rationale: High cholesterol is related to an increased LDL, VLDL, and total cholesterol. A decreased HDL can also cause hyperlipidemia. HDL is considered the "good" cholesterol, so the lower it goes, the worse the cholesterol is.

85. Which of the following lab values would most likely indicate that the patient is at an increased risk for infection?

a. **Low CD4 count**
b. High CD4 count
c. Low D-diner
d. High D-dimer

Correct Answer: A

Rationale: As HIV progresses, the CD4 count gets lower and lower without treatment. This will eventually lead to AIDS when the count gets very low (below 200). As the CD4 count drops, it increases the risk for infection. Infections and complications from AIDS are what eventually lead to death.

86. You are caring for a patient who has been admitted for a sickle cell crisis. This disorder is characterized by the abnormal appearance of the red blood cells (RBCs), most resembling which of the following shapes?

a. Square
b. Circle
c. **Crescent**
d. Oval

Correct Answer: C

Rationale: Sickle cell disease is a genetic problem in which the RBCs (red blood cells) become misshapen into a crescent like form instead of its usual round form. The crescent shape that the RBCs form resemble a sickled shape, hence the name of the disease. In this shape, it becomes difficult for the cells to pass through the capillaries. They begin to get plugged and start to build up. This can lead to very severe pain throughout the body when there is a sickle cell "crisis."

87. The doctor has ordered an arterial blood gas (ABG) to assess the patient's respiratory status. You know that a normal pH level is in which range?

a. 7.05-7.15
b. 7.35-7.45
c. 6.35-6.45
d. 7.55-7.65

Correct Answer: B

Rationale: Normal pH is in the range of 7.35 and 7.45. Acidosis can be defined as a pH below 7.35, whereas alkalosis is a pH above 7.45.

88. Which lab value would most likely be increased in the patient with congestive heart failure (CHF)?

a. **Atrial Natriuretic Peptide (ANP)**
b. Red Blood Cells (RBCs)
c. Blood Urea Nitrogen (BUN)
d. Bilirubin

Correct Answer: A

Rationale: ANP is a substance that gets sent from the atria in the heart whenever there is an increased amount of blood volume. A typical example of this would be in CHF, a condition this test is commonly used for. This main function is to lower the blood volume by decreasing water and sodium, which will eventually cause a decrease in the blood pressure.

89. A patient with liver disease is shown to have an increased bilirubin. The nurse knows that indirect bilirubin is made up of, in part, from which substance in the body?

a. White Blood Cells
b. **Hemoglobin**
c. Saliva
d. Urine

Correct Answer: B

Rationale: After hemoglobin gets released from RBCs (red blood cells), it is simplified into heme and globin. The heme eventually becomes bilirubin. This type of bilirubin is considered "Indirect." "Direct" bilirubin comes from the liver when the indirect bilirubin is linked with a substance known as a glucuronide. This direct bilirubin is then sent out to the hepatic ducts, common bile duct, and the bowel. Total bilirubin is the sum of the indirect and direct bilirubin.

90. Triglycerides are an important component when evaluating cholesterol levels. Before excess triglycerides are deposited into fatty tissue, what is their main function?

a. Fight infection
b. Store energy
c. Increase blood volume
d. Increase gastric motility

Correct Answer: B

Rationale: Triglycerides are measured, along with other labs, to determine a patient's cholesterol level and risk for other problems. They are a form of fat made in the liver and like to tag along with lipoproteins (LDLs and VLDLs). The main function of triglycerides is to store energy, but end up getting dumped into fatty tissues when there is too much of it.

91. Which of the following electrolytes is the main cation on the inside of the cells?

a. **Potassium**
b. Sodium
c. Magnesium
d. Chloride

Correct Answer: A

Rationale: Potassium is one of the most important electrolytes in the body. It plays a vital role in many functions, especially in the cardiac system. It is the main cation (positive charge) inside of the cells. However, the major effects it has are due to the concentration of potassium extracellularly (in the serum).

92. A 22 year-old male patient with type 1 diabetes was found down by a family member and is in diabetic ketoacidosis (DKA). Which of the following lab values would the nurse be most concerned with while treating this condition?

a. Hemoglobin
b. Triglycerides
c. **Anion Gap**
d. C-reactive protein

Correct Answer: C

Rationale: The anion gap is a measure of the difference between the cations (+) and the anions (-) that are in the extracellular fluid. The higher the number, the more acidotic (+) the blood is. This can happen in a few different cases, but is of special concern in lactic acidosis and diabetic ketoacidosis (DKA).

93. Which of the following lab results is a common finding in a patient with liver disease?

   a. Decreased Aspartate Aminotransferase (AST, SGOT)
   b. Decreased Prothrombin Time (PT)
   c. Increased Platelet Count (Plts)
   d. Increased Aspartate Aminotransferase (AST, SGOT)

Correct Answer: D

Rationale: Increased ALT and AST are common lab values associated with liver disease. It is doubtful that an increased platelet count would be present, as this often decreases in this situation. Prothrombin time is also typically increased, not decreased.

94. Your patient with growth hormone (GH, HGH) deficiency would like to know more about their condition. You know that growth hormone is secreted from which of the following?

a. Posterior pituitary gland
b. Adrenal glands
c. **Anterior pituitary gland**
d. Thyroid gland

Correct Answer: C

Rationale: Growth Hormone is secreted by the anterior pituitary gland. Its function does exactly what you think it does—it helps us grow. It has many other functions also, but this is the primary thing it does until the end of puberty. Sometimes, the anterior pituitary doesn't secrete enough GH, which may cause growth deficiencies and even dwarfism. If too much is secreted, you might get gigantism or acromegaly.

95. A 79-year-old female with a history of atrial flutter is admitted for possible Coumadin (warfarin) toxicity. Her gums bleed when brushing her teeth, and she now has epistaxis that she has been unable to control. Which of the following medications can be given to counteract the effects of the Coumadin?

a. **Vitamin K**
b. Potassium
c. Heparin
d. Vitamin D

Correct Answer: A

Rationale: Coumadin is an anticoagulant taken by patients who are at a high risk for blood clots (atrial fibrillation, DVT history, artificial heart valves, etc). These patients are kept at a therapeutic range, as you don't want the INR to be too high or too low. The higher the INR, the thinner the blood, and the greater the risk is for bleeding. If the INR gets too high, there are a few ways to bring it down. The first thing you will need to do is stop taking the Coumadin. You can give IV vitamin K, which is a sort of antidote to Coumadin. In a pinch, FFP (fresh frozen plasma) can be given to bring it down quickly, though it's not a long-term solution.

96. A patient who is post-op day 3 from a laparoscopic ascending colon resection has become hypotensive and tachycardic, with a fever of 102.5 F. The attending physician has ordered a lactic acid level to be drawn. Which of the following conditions is the most likely to be diagnosed if this lab value is elevated?

a. Anemia
b. Congestive heart failure
c. **Sepsis**
d. Dehydration

Correct Answer: C

Rationale: The body likes to function on aerobic metabolism, in which there is plenty of oxygen available for the tissues. In this state, glucose gets metabolized to CO_2 and H_2O. But, anaerobic metabolism happens when the amount of oxygen to the tissues decreases. Glucose then gets metabolized to lactic acid, rather than CO_2. As the lactate increases more and more, patients can develop lactic acidosis. This is something that can happen in septic shock, severe liver disease, carbon monoxide poisoning, diabetes, and with certain medications (such as metformin).

97. A patient who is 32 weeks pregnant has been admitted to the labor and delivery unit with severe preeclampsia. When medications fail to bring the blood pressure down to an acceptable level, the physician is concerned that the baby may have to be delivered early. An L/S (lecithin/sphingomyelin) ratio is ordered, a test that primarily checks for which of the following?

a. Brain maturity of the fetus
b. Heart maturity of the fetus
c. Kidney maturity of the fetus
d. **Lung maturity of the fetus**

Correct Answer: D

Rationale: The L/S Ratio is used to test how well the lungs of a fetus have matured. The sample is taken from the amniotic fluid, a process called an amniocentesis. Surfactant is a very important substance that allows the lungs to work properly, but is even more vital for premature babies. Lecithin (L) and Sphingomyelin (S) are a big part of the make-up of surfactant. This is a test that may be performed if the baby needs to be delivered pre-term.

98. Your patient with atrial fibrillation is on chronic Coumadin therapy. Which lab value would you expect to be increased because of this medication?

    a. Hematocrit
    b. Platelets
    c. Troponin
    d. INR

Correct Answer: D

Rationale: INR is used primarily to measure the effectiveness of warfarin (Coumadin), an anticoagulant taken by patients who are at a high risk for blood clots (atrial fibrillation, DVT history, artificial heart valves, etc). These patients are kept at a therapeutic range, as you don't want the INR to be too high or too low. The higher the INR, the thinner the blood, and the greater the risk is for bleeding. The lower the INR, the thicker the blood, and the greater the risk is for clotting.

99. Release of the Parathyroid hormone (PTH) can be stimulated by which of the following?

a. Low sodium
b. Low potassium
c. **Low calcium**
d. High potassium

Correct Answer: C

Rationale: When the calcium level in the body is low, the parathyroid gland responds by releasing PTH into the bloodstream. It stimulates the osteoclasts in the bone to release calcium and causes the kidneys to reabsorb it, as well as increase the absorption by the GI system.

100.   Your patient has been placed on
an IV heparin drip after being diagnosed
with a DVT in the right leg. Which of the
following lab values would be most
appropriate to monitor the effectiveness
of the heparin?

a. Thromboelastography (TEG)
b. Atrial Natriuretic Peptide (ANP)
c. Brain Natriuretic Peptide (BNP)
d. **Partial Thromboplastin Time (PTT)**

Correct Answer: D

Rationale: The PTT is one of several ways
to determine how well a patient is
coagulating, or how well an anticoagulant
is working. A common medication used
for anticoagulation is Heparin. PTT is
often used to monitor its effectiveness,
especially if it is being used as a
continuous drip. Heparin has a very quick
effect, with the PTT changing within hours
after titrating an IV drip.

101.   Which of the following lab tests would most likely indicate that liver damage is present?

a. Low Creatinine
b. **High Alanine Aminotransferase (ALT, SGPT)**
c. Low Alanine Aminotransferase (ALT, SGPT)
d. High Creatinine

Correct Answer: B

Rationale: Increased ALT and AST are common lab values associated with liver disease. Creatinine is a lab test used to measure kidney function primarily.

102.   A 48-year-old female admitted after a total knee replacement is found to have an increased alkaline phosphatase (ALP, Alk Phos). The nurse knows that this may indicate which of the following conditions? Select all that apply.

a. Hypothyroidism
b. **Liver disease**
c. **Sarcoidosis**
d. Pernicious anemia
e. Myocardial infarction
f. **Paget disease**

Correct Answer: B, C, F

Rationale: An increased ALP may be seen in patients with liver disease, Paget disease, rickets, sarcoidosis, hyperparathyroidism, and during new bone growth. ALP might be decreased in hypothyroidism, celiac disease, scurvy, malnutrition, pernicious anemia, and when there is too much B12 in the diet.

103.   You are monitoring an 84-year-old patient from an assisted living facility, who has just been admitted to the medical-surgical floor. When reviewing the lab results, you note that the albumin level is low. This would most likely indicate which of the following conditions?

a. Dehydration
b. **Malnutrition**
c. Dementia
d. Fibromyalgia

Correct Answer: B

Rationale: Albumin is commonly decreased in patients with kidney disease, liver disease, malnutrition, celiac disease, chron's disease, and during pregnancy. It can sometimes be increased when taking certain medications and in dehydration.

104.   While treating a patient in diabetic ketoacidosis (DKA), you are unable to find the anion gap in the lab report. What is one way to calculate the anion gap using other lab values?

a. Chloride – (sodium + bicarbonate)
b. Troponin + (Creatinine – BUN)
c. Hemoglobin - hematocrit
d. **Sodium – (chloride + bicarbonate)**

Correct Answer: D

Rationale: The quickest way to determine the anion gap is to add the chloride and bicarbonate values together, then subtract this number from the sodium level. If you know the potassium level, you can be more precise. Then you would add the potassium level to the sodium level before doing the subtraction.

105.   The patient has increased amylase and lipase levels. The nurse is aware that the following condition is most likely to result in this finding:

a. **Pancreatitis**
b. Cardiomyopathy
c. Nephritis
d. Diverticulitis

Correct Answer: A

Rationale: Amylase and lipase are lab values commonly used to evaluate pancreas function. If pancreatitis is present, then these would most likely be increased.

106.   You are caring for a 47-year-old male with end-stage renal disease, on hemodialysis 3 days a week. When you look at the monitor, you notice that he is in normal sinus rhythm, but the T waves are much higher than normal (peaked). Which of the following lab values is the most likely cause for this reading?

a.   Hypokalemia
b.   Hyponatremia
c.   **Hyperkalemia**
d.   Hypernatremia

Correct Answer: C

Rationale: A cardinal sign of hyperkalemia is a peaked T wave (higher than usual) on the EKG tracing. You can also see arrhythmias, a widened QRS segment and the ST segment might be depressed. Patients may feel irritable, nauseous, or have diarrhea.

107.   Which of the following lab values would you expect to see included in a complete blood count (CBC)?

a. Glucose
b. **Hematocrit**
c. Alanine aminotransferase (ALT)
d. Lipase

Correct Answer: B

Rationale: A complete blood count (CBC) includes the white blood count (WBC), hemoglobin, hematocrit, and the platelet count.

108. The nurse is assessing a patient with Addison Disease. Which of the following areas of the body is responsible for releasing Adrenocorticotropic Hormone (ACTH)?

a. Posterior pituitary gland
b. Thymus
c. Pineal gland
d. Anterior pituitary gland

Correct Answer: D

Rationale: The ACTH measures the function of the anterior pituitary gland. Corticotropin-releasing hormone (CRH) comes from the hypothalamus and causes ACTH to be released from the anterior pituitary. Once this happens, the ACTH causes cortisol production from the adrenal cortex.

109.   Your patient with alcoholic cirrhosis is becoming progressively confused and somnolent. The doctor on call has ordered lactulose to be started immediately. Which lab value would you most likely expect to be increased in this scenario?

a. Creatinine
b. Hematocrit
c. Platelets
d. **Ammonia**

Correct Answer: D

Rationale: When a patient has severe liver problems, such as cirrhosis or hepatitis, ammonia levels can increase to dangerous levels. Normally, proteins in the body are broken down into ammonia, among other things. Ammonia then goes to the liver, which converts it into urea. The urea then goes to the kidneys and is banished from the body through the urine. When there are liver problems, this process is disrupted, and ammonia is allowed to run wild. This is not good, as it easily makes its way to the brain, causing hepatic encephalopathy. The patient might start out being confused and disoriented. If the ammonia levels continue to rise, it may eventually lead to a coma. Lactulose is a medication that be given orally or rectally to help bring down these high levels. The ammonia can then be removed by way of the colon.

110.   Red blood cells (RBCs) are a vital component to the function of the body. The nurse knows that they are produced in which of the following?

a. Smooth muscle
b. **Bone marrow**
c. Small intestine
d. Skeletal muscle

Correct Answer: B

Rationale: RBCs are produced in the bone marrow and contain hemoglobin molecules that transport oxygen and carbon dioxide throughout the body. When there are no problems present, a red blood cell can typically survive for 120 days. Rarely is the RBC count looked at on its own. It is usually compared and evaluated with the hemoglobin, hematocrit, and platelet count.

I hope you did well on the practice test! If not, no big deal. Don't give up, and I promise, you will get there!

Don't forget to leave a review on Amazon...it is very much appreciated!

Check out the web site for articles, nursing humor, and more!

www.kickassnursing.com

Made in the USA
Monee, IL
11 December 2020

52246128R00177